HEALTHCARE STRATEGIC PLANNING

THIRD EDITION

HEALTHCARE STRATEGIC PLANNING

THIRD EDITION

Alan M. Zuckerman, FACHE, FAAHC

ACHE Management Series

Your board, staff, or clients may also benefit from this book's insight. For more information on quantity discounts, contact the Health Administration Press Marketing Manager at (312) 424–9470.

Reprinted November 2014

Library of Congress Cataloging-in-Publication Data

Zuckerman, Alan M.
  Healthcare strategic planning / Alan M. Zuckerman. -- 3rd ed.
     p. ; cm. -- (ACHE management series)
  Includes bibliographical references and index.
  ISBN 978-1-56793-434-2 (alk. paper)
  I. Title. II. Series: Management series (Ann Arbor, Mich.)
  [DNLM: 1. Hospital Administration. 2. Health Planning. 3. Planning Techniques. WX 150.1]

   362.11068--dc23

                        2011051586

The paper used in this publication meets the minimum requirements of American National Standard for Information Sciences—Permanence of Paper for Printed Library Materials, ANSI Z39.48-1984. ♾ ™

Acquisitions editor: Janet Davis; Project manager: Eduard Avis; Cover designer: Gloria Chantell; Layout: Virginia Byrne

Found an error or a typo? We want to know! Please e-mail it to hap1@ache.org, and put "Book Error" in the subject line.

For photocopying and copyright information, please contact Copyright Clearance Center at www.copyright.com or at (978) 750–8400.

Health Administration Press
A division of the Foundation of the American
   College of Healthcare Executives
One North Franklin Street, Suite 1700
Chicago, IL 60606–3529
(312) 424–2800

Contents

Acknowledgments

I hope you enjoy the third edition of *Healthcare Strategic Planning* as much as I enjoyed writing it. I appreciate all of the suggestions and ideas given to me over the past six years by my clients, students in my ACHE courses, and colleagues. As a result of their input, this new edition is a much better guide to healthcare strategic planning.

There are three groups I would particularly like to acknowledge for their contributions to this third edition. First of all are my clients from the past six years, and especially those organizations that generously allowed me to share aspects of their strategic plans and processes with the field. They include the following:

- AtlantiCare, Egg Harbor Township, New Jersey
- Barnes-Jewish Hospital, St. Louis, Missouri

- British Columbia Children's Hospital, Vancouver, British Columbia
- Commonwealth Medicine/University of Massachusetts Medical School, Worcester, Massachusetts
- Health First, Inc., Melbourne, Florida
- High Point Regional Health System, High Point, North Carolina
- Hunterdon Healthcare System, Flemington, New Jersey
- Memorial Health System, Springfield, Illinois
- TriHealth, Cincinnati, Ohio
- UCSD Health System, San Diego, California
- UW Health, Madison, Wisconsin
- Wayne Memorial Health System, Wayne, Pennsylvania

Second are my colleagues at our consulting firm, Health Strategies & Solutions, Inc. Particular kudos go to Susan Arnold, marketing director, who, as before, shepherded the project from start to finish, and to Kelly Raible, marketing manager, who was a jack-of-all-trades in researching, editing, formatting, and any other task she was asked to do to get the job done.

The third group is, of course, my family, for allowing me to spend so much time on this and other "volunteer" activities. Thanks to my wife, Rita, especially. My children, Seth and Joanna, who suffered through the writing of editions one and two when they needed me to play, chauffeur, help with homework, or cook, are now on their own and didn't have much input this time, except for an occasional smart remark. But, interestingly, both have found my expertise in strategic planning useful now that they are out in the real world, so have a new understanding of the value of this work that many of you have already realized.

Alan M. Zuckerman
Philadelphia, Pennsylvania
August 2011

Preface

The first edition of *Healthcare Strategic Planning*, published in 1998, was my first foray into book publishing. My subsequent books, while modestly successful, did not make the cut for second editions. Upon reflection, I believe this is a testament to the staying power and relevancy of the topic of healthcare strategic planning and the need for a practical, how-to book that leads readers through the strategic planning process.

I have been pleased and a bit overwhelmed by the response of healthcare professionals to this book. The tools, tips, and examples from healthcare organizations that face similar pitfalls and opportunities when planning for the future have resonated with leaders in the field who are in the midst of the most transformational change ever experienced by the US healthcare delivery system. Many have shared examples of how the book helped them personally and how it impacted their organizations. A number have suggested improvements based on their own experiences.

So as I approached the writing of this third edition, I had ample material for improving upon earlier editions by sharing new research and contemporary tools and examples that should appeal to all healthcare organizations—whether their needs are strategic fine tuning or major overhauls in strategic direction. This third edition of *Healthcare Strategic Planning* is truly new and improved. I hope it will be as useful and helpful to the field as the first and second editions were.

What has been retained in the third edition is the basic structure of the recommended strategic planning approach. Chapters 3 through 6, which review each component of the strategic planning process, and chapters 2 and 7, which address preplanning preparation and planning process issues, present significant and important new material.

Here is a summary of the new material in each chapter:

- *Chapter 1—Is Strategic Planning Still Relevant?* This chapter includes new research and thinking about strategic planning within and outside of healthcare. New exhibits are presented as well, including a nonlinear strategic planning process approach.
- *Chapter 2—Organizing for Successful Strategic Planning: 12 Critical Steps.* This chapter presents new potential objectives for strategic planning that reflect the rapidly changing market conditions being experienced nationwide.
- *Chapter 3—Activity I: Analyzing the Environment.* A number of exhibits and examples have been added and updated to better illustrate the intricacies of the environmental assessment.
- *Chapter 4—Activity II: Identifying Organizational Direction.* All of the examples of mission, vision, strategy, and values statements have been updated and improved, and the guidance material about how to develop these statements has been reshaped, sharpened, and expanded.

- *Chapter 5—Activity III: Formulating Strategy.* Many new and revised examples and tools are included in this chapter along with a new section on contingency planning.
- *Chapter 6—Activity IV: Transitioning to Implementation.* The transition from planning to implementation has proven to be a difficult task for many organizations. Specific guidance on this topic is provided in this chapter, including a strategic plan summary example that includes pillars of excellence, an implementation plan format, transition management guidelines, and ideas for communicating and rolling out the plan's findings and recommendations to stakeholders.
- *Chapter 7—Major Planning Process Considerations.* Additional guidance on research approaches is presented, and new material on how to advance the planning process to the next level, including process improvement tips and bottom-up planning, has been incorporated.
- *Chapter 8—Realizing Benefits from Strategic Planning.* This chapter argues that strategic planning needs to produce tangible, important benefits to remain relevant and suggests that most healthcare organizations should attempt to realize benefits in four broad categories: products/markets, finances, operations, and community health.
- *Chapter 9—Making Planning Stick: From Implementation to Managing Strategically.* Several new exhibits present contemporary thinking about barriers to strategy execution, a concise overview of ongoing strategic planning activities, and an action plan progress review example.
- *Chapter 10—The Annual Strategic Plan Update.* Many healthcare organizations conduct an annual planning update. This topic, only briefly discussed in the first edition, is expanded in the third edition with new case studies of Commonwealth Medicine and AtlantiCare.
- *Chapter 11—Encouraging Strategic Thinking.* Substantial new material on strategic thinking has been added as this concept

continues to garner interest within and outside of healthcare. The red ocean and blue ocean concepts are examined in detail.

* *Chapter 12—Future Challenges for Strategic Planning and Planners.* A new section in this chapter describes the five qualities of planning practices at pathbreaking companies outside of healthcare.

For instructors who use this book in their classes, all exhibits from the book are available on PowerPoint slides. For access, please write to hap1@ache.org.

Ad hoc planning, educated guesses, and intuition have allowed some organizations to survive, although many have now succumbed to the current wave of hospital and system consolidation and closure. These approaches alone will not serve healthcare organizations well as they contend with an increasingly competitive and financially unstable operating environment and the still uncertain impact of healthcare reform initiatives. I fervently believe that planning that is truly strategic—envisioning a desired future that may challenge conventions and then crafting creative and groundbreaking strategies that will take organizations there—will distinguish those providers at risk for closure from those that will thrive. I hope this book will be a call to action for healthcare executives and will inspire and motivate them to use strategic planning to lead their organizations into a new era of serving the healthcare needs of their communities.

Alan M. Zuckerman
Philadelphia, Pennsylvania
August 2011

CHAPTER 1

Is Strategic Planning Still Relevant?

Planning is bringing the future into the present so that you can do something about it now.

—*Alan Lakein*

If you don't know where you're going, any road will take you there.

—*Lewis Carroll*

Strategic planning has been an important and frequently used management tool, both inside and outside of healthcare, for decades; however, questions about its relevancy and effectiveness in that role have persisted.

Swayne, Duncan, and Ginter (2008) note that "After almost four decades of research, the effects of strategic planning on an organization's performance are still unclear. Some studies have found significant benefits from planning, although others have found no relationship, or even small negative effects."

While academicians and industry analysts are divided on the bottom-line value of strategic planning, executives and managers on the front lines argue that it is still relevant and even consider it a central management and governance discipline, especially in rapidly changing operating environments. Bellenfant and Nelson

(2010) write, "Those organizations that look to the future, by planning and evolving to meet expected changes head on, will have a better chance of survival. Strategic planning has added value to hospitals that are looking for ways to protect their financial viability while adapting to the ever-changing environment around them." While Begun and Kaissi (2005) confirm that little is known about the extent to which healthcare organizations conduct formal strategic planning or how it affects performance, their study of 20 healthcare organizations indicates that strategic planning is a common and valued function. Most of the leaders at the organizations studied responded that strategic planning contributes to organizational focus, fosters stakeholder participation and commitment, and leads to achievement of strategic goals.

A 2005 survey of 440 provider-based healthcare professionals found that strategic planning is practiced with regularity by healthcare organizations and appears to be a well-regarded process among executives (Zuckerman 2007). Nearly 40 percent of respondents developed or updated their strategic plans annually, and another 40 percent did so every two to three years. On a five-point scale, with five being the highest rating and one the lowest, questions asking respondents to rate their strategic planning processes and outcomes received an average response of nearly four.

STRATEGIC PLANNING IS...

The concept of strategy has roots in both political and military history, from Sun Tzu to Homer and Euripides (Swayne, Duncan, and Ginter 2008). The word *strategy* comes from the Greek *stratego*, which means "to plan the destruction of one's enemies through effective use of resources" (Bracker 1980). Many terms associated with strategic planning, such as *objective, mission, strength*, and *weakness*, were developed by or used in the military (Swayne, Duncan, and Ginter 2008).

A number of definitions have evolved to pinpoint the essence of strategic planning. According to Swayne, Duncan, and Ginter (2008), "strategic planning defines where the organization is going, sometimes where it is not going, and provides focus. The plan sets direction for the organization and—through a common understanding of the vision and broad strategic goals—provides a template for everyone in the organization to make consistent decisions that move the organization toward its envisioned future. Strategic planning, in large part, is a decision-making activity."

Beckham (2000) describes true strategy as "a plan for getting from a point in the present to some point in the future in the face of uncertainty and resistance." Campbell (1993) adds the concept of measurement to his definition: "Strategic planning refers to a process for defining organizational objectives, implementing strategies to achieve those objectives, and measuring the effectiveness of those strategies."

Evashwick and Evashwick (1988), incorporating the concepts of vision and mission, define strategic planning as "the process for assessing a changing environment to create a vision of the future; determining how the organization fits into the anticipated environment based on its institutional mission, strengths, and weaknesses; and then setting in motion a plan of action to position the organization accordingly."

STRATEGIC PLANNING OUTSIDE OF HEALTHCARE

Strategic planning has been used in the general business community since the mid-twentieth century. Planning, programming, and budgeting systems were introduced in the late 1940s and early 1950s but used only sparingly by business and government at that time. In the 1960s and 1970s, leading firms such as General Electric practiced strategic planning, promoting the merits of providing a framework beyond the 12-month cycle and a systematic approach to managing business units (Webster, Reif, and Bracker 1989).

Strategic planning in the 1980s and 1990s was based on corporate market planning, which emphasizes maximizing profits through identification of a market segment and development of strategies to control that segment (Spiegel and Hyman 1991). An emphasis on total quality management and productivity also emerged in strategic planning in the 1980s as strategists followed the lead of Jack Welch, head of General Electric.

In the twenty-first century, competitive strategy has become a prominent feature in strategic planning practices, along with a notable uptick in plans that call for alliances and mergers. But today's profoundly uncertain times have forced business strategists to acknowledge that strategic planning as usual will not provide the foundation needed to survive tumultuous economic conditions. Dye, Sibony, and Viguerie (2009) note that scenario planning, a tested technique for coping with uncertainty, will play a more critical role in strategic planning and companies must consider more variables and involve more decision makers than in the past. They also predict that greater emphasis on measurement will be needed to monitor changing market conditions and make quick strategic adjustments.

Rheault (2003) contends that quick reactions are valued more than well-reasoned responses in highly dynamic markets, but Einblau (2003) points out that change is inevitable—sometimes it happens quickly and other times it evolves slowly, but it always happens.

Our external environment is one of market uncertainty, international political unrest, and shifting social values; current economic imbalances will continue to occur and will continue to be managed. Operating in this uncertain climate requires that we envision our desired future and then plan the strategies needed to get us there; otherwise we will always be accepting the future someone else has worked to make happen, and in business, that someone else is usually a competitor.

An irony noted by Hamel (1996) is that most strategic planning is not strategic. He stresses that only a small portion of an industry's conventions is ever challenged and that the planning processes harness only a small amount of an organization's creative potential. Hamel suggests that most strategy planning can be characterized as ritualistic, reductionist, extrapolative, positioning, and elitist. Instead, he says, strategic planning should be inquisitive, expansive, prescient, inventive, inclusive, and demanding. Hamel also emphasizes that strategy making is assumed to be easy, which of course it is if organizations limit the scope of discovery, the breadth of involvement, and the amount of intellectual effort expended.

A 2006 *McKinsey Quarterly* survey of almost 800 business executives found that while three-quarters of the respondents reported that their company had a formal strategic planning process, fewer than half were satisfied with their company's approach to planning strategy. The most significant concerns focused on executing the strategy, communicating it, aligning the organization with the strategy, and measuring performance against the plan (McKinsey 2006).

Despite the uncertainties about its value, strategic planning is being used frequently and is considered critical to the success of organizations. A 2003 survey by the Buttonwood Group of 225 US companies (the average company having more than 3,000 employees and $850 million in sales) revealed that the annual strategic plan required 10.5 days of work for about 22 percent of that company's employees. The average company represented in the survey spent $3.1 million to produce the plan (Taub 2003).

HEALTHCARE STRATEGIC PLANNING

Healthcare organizations have used strategic planning sporadically since the 1970s, orienting it toward providing services and meeting the needs of the population. Prior to the 1970s, healthcare organizations were predominately independent and not-for-profit, and healthcare planning was usually conducted on a local or regional basis by state, county, or municipal governments.

Exhibit 1.1: Healthcare Strategic Planning: A History

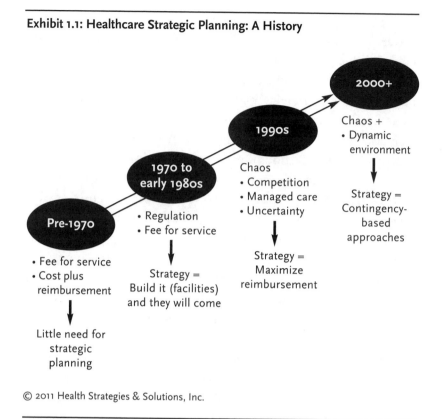

© 2011 Health Strategies & Solutions, Inc.

As illustrated in Exhibit 1.1, from the 1970s through the early 1980s, regulation became more prominent, but the fee-for-service system ensured steady revenue sources. When healthcare organizations engaged in strategic planning, the effort often focused on facilities, with the prevailing notion that "if you build it, they will come." The 1990s were characterized by the chaos generated from the emergence of managed care and competition among providers who had previously been collegial. Strategic planning conducted in that decade featured a heavy emphasis on maximizing reimbursement.

Chaos is still evident in twenty-first-century healthcare organizations as they continue to contend with competition and reimbursement issues and the added challenge of an increasingly dynamic environment. The Patient Protection and Affordable Care Act, signed into law in March 2010 and preceded by many months of speculation about what the legislation might include, has ushered in a new era of strategic planning. Providers across the country are examining their current and future role in an era of reform where quality, service, cost competitiveness, scale and scope, and integration will move to the forefront of strategic priorities.

For many healthcare organizations, previously crafted strategies must be reexamined, and in some cases, a strategic overhaul may be needed to orient the organization to the realities of the reformed marketplace. Providers are being challenged to focus on improving their market positions and increasingly differentiate themselves from the competition in their key service lines. Merger or acquisition strategies are prominent nationwide, particularly so in crowded markets and those with financially fragile healthcare organizations.

Rapidly changing technology; increasing competition from physician entrepreneurs and for-profit niche providers; and the looming shortage of physicians, nurses, and other healthcare professionals will also contribute an element of uncertainty to the healthcare environment. Healthcare organizations with comprehensive, sound strategic plans will be best positioned to respond with contingency plans as change emerges.

The Strategic Planning Process

Many variations of a strategic planning model have emerged in the business and healthcare communities, but the basic model remains relatively unchanged. Two similar approaches to strategic planning were developed in the 1980s. The first, documented by Sorkin, Ferris, and Hudak (1984) features the following steps:

- Scan the environment
- Select key issues

- Set a mission statement and broad goals
- Undertake external and internal analyses
- Develop goals, objectives, and strategies for each issue
- Develop an implementation plan to carry out strategic actions
- Monitor, update, and scan

The second was tailored to healthcare and included these steps (Simyar, Lloyd-Jones, and Caro 1988):

- Identify the organization's current position, including present mission, long-term objectives, strategies, and policies
- Analyze the environment
- Conduct an organizational audit
- Identify the various alternative strategies based on relevant data
- Select the best alternative
- Gain acceptance
- Prepare long-range and short-range plans to support and carry out the strategy
- Implement the plan and conduct an ongoing evaluation

For the purposes of this book, the steps from the two approaches are synthesized into four stages, as illustrated in Exhibit 1.2. The first stage is the environmental assessment, which focuses on the question, Where are we now? It includes four activities:

1. Organizational review, including mission, philosophy, and culture
2. External assessment
3. Internal assessment
4. Evaluation of competitive position, including advantages and disadvantages

Exhibit 1.2: The Strategic Planning Approach

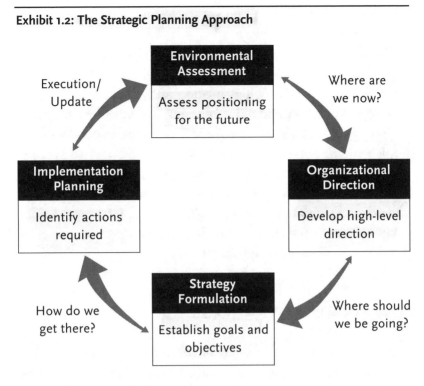

© 2011 Health Strategies & Solutions, Inc.

The goal of environmental assessments is to determine how external forces might affect the organization in the future and what factors might be addressed to deal with environmental challenges.

The second stage of the planning process is organizational direction, followed by the third stage, strategy formulation. Stages two and three address the question, Where should we be going? The main activity of the organizational direction stage is to develop a future strategic profile by examining alternative futures, mission, vision, values, and key strategies for the organization. Strategy formulation establishes goals, objectives, and major initiatives for the organization. The purpose of stages two and three of the planning process is to determine what broad, future direction is possible and desirable and what future scope of services and position the organization will strive to achieve.

The fourth stage is implementation planning—How do we get there? This stage involves identifying the actions needed to implement the plan. Key activities include mapping out the tasks to accomplish the goals and objectives, setting a schedule, determining priorities, and allocating resources to ensure implementation. Implementation should occur as soon as possible after completion of the plan, if not during the final stage. Commitment to ongoing monitoring of plan implementation and completion of periodic updates and revisions, as needed, should be in place prior to finalizing the plan. Each stage of the planning process is discussed in detail in the following chapters.

WHY STRATEGIC PLANNING?

The pervasive and deep impact of environmental change on healthcare providers may lead some healthcare executives and boards to conclude that long-term planning is a pointless exercise. Could ad hoc planning be as effective as a long-term strategic plan that is crafted during a period of rapid change and uncertainty? Healthcare organizations have historically survived using less formalized planning approaches.

Despite uncertain market conditions and unstable economic circumstances, healthcare providers can rely on a number of certainties. Regardless of whether healthcare reform is repealed, altered, or left as is, healthcare organizations will have to do more with less. Value will be the hallmark of successful providers. The population will continue to age. Patient care that is coordinated and of the highest quality will be rewarded. The shortage of physicians, nurses, and other care professionals will not go away. Failing to plan for these inevitabilities and others or postponing action to mitigate them could weaken a healthcare organization to the point where survival is not possible.

THE BENEFITS OF STRATEGIC PLANNING

Fogg (1994) suggests the following benefits of strategic planning:

- It **secures the future** for the organization and its leaders by crafting a viable future business.
- It **provides a road map, direction, and focus** for the organization's future—where it wants to go and the routes to get there. It lets each part of the organization align its activities with the direction of the corporation in a continuous process.
- It **sets priorities** for the crucial strategic tasks, including the complex, burning issues such as lack of direction and growth, lack of profitability, and organizational ineffectiveness that everybody talks and knows about while wondering why they are not being addressed.
- It **allocates resources** available for growth and change to the programs and activities with the highest potential payoff.
- It **establishes measures** of success so that the progress of the organization and individuals can be gauged. Knowing where one stands is a fundamental business and human need.
- It **gathers input and ideas** from all parts of the organization on what can be done to ensure future success and eliminate barriers to that success, following the old adage that ten or one hundred or one thousand heads are better than one.
- It **generates commitment** to implement the plan by involving all parts of the organization in its development.
- It **coordinates** the actions of diverse and separate parts of the organization into unified programs to accomplish objectives.

Fogg (1994) further notes that

When all is said and done, employees also recognize what's in it for them personally: the resources to do what they want if they plan; a more secure future if the organization plans well and does well;

financial rewards if they make themselves heroes as a result of the process; recognition by their peers and superiors if they succeed; and, of course, the inverse of all the above if they fail.

Swayne, Duncan, and Ginter (2008) believe that the three stages of strategic management—strategic thinking, strategic planning, and strategic momentum—provide many benefits, including

- tying the organization together with a common sense of purpose and shared values;
- improving financial performance in many cases;
- providing the organization with a clear self-concept, specific goals, and guidance and consistency in decision making;
- helping managers understand the present, think about the future, and recognize the signals that suggest change;
- requiring managers to communicate both vertically and horizontally;
- improving overall coordination within the organization; and
- encouraging innovation and change within the organization to meet the needs of dynamic situations.

According to Nadler (1994), for many organizations the true value of strategic planning lies in the process, not the plan. "Most plans have a tremendously fast rate of depreciation. By the time they're printed and bound they've become obsolete. The value of planning is largely in the shared learning, the shared frame of reference, the shared context for those small decisions that get made over time."

Indeed, changes that influence a strategic plan may occur daily, and new ideas may surface once the plan is complete. A successful strategic plan enables providers to establish a consistent, articulated direction for the future. But it is also a living document that must be monitored and revised to meet anticipated and unanticipated needs of the organization and the market, whether changes occur in managed care, integrated delivery, healthcare reform, systems development, technological advances, or other arenas.

WHAT IS EFFECTIVE STRATEGY?

Beckham (2000) proposes seven key characteristics of effective strategy:

1. **Sustainability**. It has lasting power with greater long-term impact than other initiatives.
2. **Performance improvement**. It results in significant improvement in key performance indicators.
3. **Quality**. It is a demonstrably superior approach to those of competitors.
4. **Direction**. It moves the organization toward a defined end, although not necessarily in a linear fashion.
5. **Focus**. It is targeted and represents a choice to pursue a certain course over other attractive alternatives.
6. **Connection**. Its components have a high level of interdependence and synergy.
7. **Importance**. It may not be essential to organizational success, but it is certainly significant or fundamental.

"must be measurable"

   Healthcare organizations undertake considerable strategic planning and strategizing, yet much of this effort fails to achieve the benefits and outcomes cited in this chapter, and sometimes it is completely ineffective. Senior leaders can increase the value of their strategic planning by measuring the performance of the organization's strategy against Beckham's seven characteristics and avoiding many of the problems described in the next section.

TYPICAL PROBLEMS THAT LIMIT THE EFFECTIVENESS OF STRATEGIC PLANNING

Many healthcare organizations that undertake strategic planning experience common problems that leave their leaders jaded about the value of such planning.

Failing to Involve the Appropriate People

Sometimes too many stakeholders are involved; sometimes too few are. Sometimes, the number of participants is fine but those involved are not necessarily the "right" people. Thoughtful involvement of the right type and mix of internal and external stakeholders is essential.

Conducting Strategic Planning Independently of Financial Planning

If financial considerations are excluded from the strategic plan, strategies may never become a reality. Sound strategic planning will explicitly incorporate financial realities and capabilities.

Falling Prey to Analysis Paralysis

The fast-paced healthcare market demands that providers respond to opportunities and threats without extensive delays. Many providers are lulled into a sense of security when they are planning and squander time over endless fine-tuning and revisions. When exhaustive planning takes over, very little change or progress occurs.

Not Addressing the Critical Issues

The most pressing issues may not be addressed because they are too difficult to deal with or so many issues are identified that none are appropriately addressed. If leadership is not prepared to initiate discussions of key issues, strategic plans focus on minor topics and ignore the most critical and threatening challenges.

Assuming that Established Objectives Take Care of Themselves

Failure to implement a strategic plan is one of the most common flaws of the planning process. Staff may be overwhelmed with managing day-to-day crises, leaving little time to implement strategic objectives. The objectives may also lack precision, so that ensuing activities lack direction.

Failing to Achieve Consensus

Even a great strategic plan cannot succeed without strong support and enthusiasm. Leadership must garner support directly from stakeholders to ensure that the benefits of the strategic plan are realized.

Lacking Flexibility and Responsiveness to the Dynamic Environment

Plans can be too rigid, inhibiting flexibility, creativity, and innovation. A more fluid, dynamic, and ongoing process, as suggested in the strategic management approach described in Chapter 9, should help address this issue.

Ignoring Resistance to Change

Resistance to change can cause delays, waste, or complete derailment of a strategic priority. Failure to address resistance swiftly and directly may lead to chronic and long-term consequences with devastating effects.

CONCLUSION

When strategic planning first became commonplace in health-care in the early to mid 1980s, it was a first-generation approach applied in a far less complex healthcare environment than we operate in today. Thirty years later, state-of-the-art strategic planning has become much more sophisticated, driven by improvements in related disciplines and developments in the field.

Strategic planning's application in healthcare organizations today differs from that of the past in five critical ways:

1. **The environment has evolved and is changing at an even faster pace.** The rate of change is a key factor in causing strategic planning to be practiced in a more dynamic fashion.
2. **The competitive environment is much more intense than at any time in the past.** The number of competitors, the increasing for-profit influence in healthcare delivery, the decline of geographic barriers to competition as a result of the Internet, and other less significant factors raise the competitive stakes and force strategic planning to be more externally focused and fluid.
3. **Healthcare organizations have grown into vast multientity systems.** The emergence of systems, especially in the past five to ten years, has ratcheted up the complexity of strategic planning.
4. **The financial underpinning of healthcare delivery has been destabilized.** When organizations are operating in an environment of increasing financial risk and uncertainty, strategic planning needs to be linked more clearly to financial planning and contribute more directly to financial performance.

5. **The time frame within which to act and generate results is increasingly shortened.** Strategic planning must address near-term pressures while still directing organizations toward long-term targets.

With this chapter as a backdrop, succeeding chapters present contemporary strategic planning approaches.

CHAPTER 2

Organizing for Successful Strategic Planning: 12 Critical Steps

Organizing is what you do before you do something, so that when you do it, it is not all mixed up.

—A. A. Milne

By failing to prepare, you are preparing to fail.

—Benjamin Franklin

In the early stages of writing the first edition of this book, I omitted this chapter. Instead, I chose to dive into the topic of performing the actual work of strategic planning and began to describe its process and products. However, as I tried to describe what must be accomplished in strategic planning and why, I realized I had left out the first, most critical activity: organizing for successful strategic planning.

Looking back on the hundreds of strategic plans I have reviewed, and the many planning and management staffs I have spoken with about strategic planning, I see that one common mistake made in an organization's strategic planning process is the failure to organize before beginning the so-called real work of strategic planning. To avoid this pitfall, the following 12 steps should be completed in advance of strategic planning:

1. Identify and communicate strategic planning objectives
2. Describe and communicate the planning process
3. Assert CEO leadership of strategic planning
4. Define and communicate the roles and responsibilities of other organizational leaders
5. Identify the strategic planning facilitator
6. Establish and communicate the strategic planning schedule
7. Assemble relevant historical data
8. Resolve not to overanalyze historical data
9. Review past strategies and identify successes and failures
10. Conduct strategic planning orientation meetings
11. Prepare to stimulate new thinking
12. Reinforce future orientation

IDENTIFY AND COMMUNICATE STRATEGIC PLANNING OUTCOMES

The word *communicate* is integral to the first six steps of organizing for strategic planning. One common mistake made in traditional healthcare strategic planning is that too few people undertake too much analysis. The planning process should include as many elements of organizational leadership and as many different perspectives as possible. To ensure widespread participation, emphasize communication of strategic planning objectives to the entire healthcare organization from the outset of the organizational phase.

The importance of clear outcomes to successful strategic planning cannot be overstated. General outcomes-oriented statements such as "Strategic planning will provide our organization with a road map for the future" or "Strategic planning will allow our organization to allocate scarce resources in the most effective manner possible" are not specific enough to prove to all constituencies that expending time and resources for strategic planning is worthwhile.

Specific strategic planning objectives should be established and reviewed periodically during the planning process to ensure that priority issues are being addressed and that the plan is on track to produce outputs that satisfy these objectives. Some specific objectives for the healthcare delivery environment of the twenty-first century include determining how to

- prepare for and respond to market consolidation and increasing competitive pressures;
- achieve the highest quality and best outcomes at the lowest cost;
- coordinate and integrate care with physicians and nonacute care providers;
- increase access to services, especially primary and preventive care;
- respond to demands for consumer-driven healthcare, including patient-centric care and increased availability and transparency of information; and
- address the shortage of physicians, nurses, and other healthcare professionals.

DESCRIBE AND COMMUNICATE THE PLANNING PROCESS

Too often, planning begins without a clear sense of what the planning process entails. In these cases, planning may commence as a reaction to questions raised by the organization's board or senior management. As these leaders deliberate their answers, they decide that the best context in which to deliver them is an as-yet-unspecified strategic planning process. Thus, migration into what is called strategic planning begins without a careful and thoughtful attempt to understand why or how planning should occur.

Whether your organization chooses the strategic planning process described in this book or one from the abundance of other available materials on the subject, it is imperative to identify and customize it to meet the organization's specific needs prior to initiating strategic planning. Once a process is developed to meet the specific strategic planning objectives of the organization, it must be communicated effectively to organizational leadership and other important stakeholders. Leadership and stakeholders will feel removed from the strategic planning, be reluctant to participate, or participate ineffectively if they lack understanding of the process.

ASSERT CEO LEADERSHIP OF STRATEGIC PLANNING

In nearly all organizations, including healthcare organizations, the CEO leads the strategic planning process. Other people may also play important roles, and in a not-for-profit organization the board of directors is especially critical. However, the CEO should be the leader.

Fogg (1994) suggests that at the outset of the planning process, the following key aspects of the CEO's role and leadership responsibilities be clarified and communicated:

- Demonstrate and continually reinforce the importance of planning in the organization
- Allocate time, money, staff support, and personal support to the planning process
- Set high standards for the planning process and results
- Encourage creativity and the search for the unlikely or not so obvious
- Lead the development of an inspired, comprehensive, and far-reaching vision for the organization
- Make, push, or affirm timely decisions
- Serve as the principal link between the planning process and important external constituencies
- Hold senior staff and others accountable for results and reward them accordingly
- Install an ongoing integrated planning process and infrastructure

By asserting a strong presence at the start of the strategic planning process and then executing key elements of the leadership role throughout it, the CEO appears, appropriately, as the champion of strategic planning and increases the probability of a smoothly functioning process and successful results.

DEFINE AND COMMUNICATE THE ROLES AND RESPONSIBILITIES OF OTHER ORGANIZATIONAL LEADERS

Strategic planning is a major responsibility of a board, particularly in not-for-profit organizations. The board represents the community, which in not-for-profits is the owner of the organization. As such, the board needs to play an especially significant role in setting and guarding the mission and values of the organization. It also should serve as a key adviser to staff on other significant plan elements. And ultimately, it is the board that must approve or reject the strategic plan.

In healthcare organizations, strategic planning is a mechanism for bringing physicians—whether employed by the organization or not—into the process of collectively determining the future direction of the organization and its related entities, such as physician groups. Depending on the nature of the organization, other clinicians may also play a key role in strategic planning.

Commentators in the literature differ in their opinion of how important it is for various organizational constituencies to participate in the strategic planning process, and of how broad and deep that involvement should be. Some experts believe that executive management is principally responsible for planning and that other stakeholders' involvement should be limited. Some believe that the best plans are developed when stakeholders in the organization participate broadly and frequently. The perspective espoused in this book falls closer to the latter view. Chapter 7 discusses this issue further.

Here, as in the planning preparation steps discussed earlier, there is no single answer for every organization, but rather a choice to be made, typically by the CEO and senior management team, from among available alternatives. Regardless of the level of participation selected, the decision should be made before the planning process begins and be communicated clearly to all affected constituencies. Once the strategic planning process is formally initiated, board members, management staff, physicians, and others will understand their roles in the planning process and what specific responsibilities they will have as it unfolds.

In most healthcare organizations, a strategic planning committee is established to oversee the planning process. This group may be a standing committee of the board or created to serve on an ad hoc basis. Initially, the committee should aim to

- describe and discuss strategic planning outcomes;
- review and revise the strategic planning approach and schedule, including identification of key project meetings and other milestones;
- review the initial database and identify sources for any additional data required;
- identify internal and external stakeholders to be interviewed;
- identify other primary market research to be conducted, including intended audiences and purpose of market research; and
- discuss the mechanisms for interface among the planning staff, external advisers (as applicable), and the organization, including
  1. staff contacts for logistical support;
  2. interaction with the board, medical staff, and other constituents; and
  3. logistical issues related to the planning process.

IDENTIFY THE STRATEGIC PLANNING FACILITATOR

While the CEO may be the leader of strategic planning, day-to-day facilitation of the process is typically managed by another individual. How facilitation will be carried out must be resolved at the outset of the process.

Fogg (1994) suggests that

> Most CEOs depend upon a skilled, objective strategic planning facilitator to jump-start the organization into strategic planning and to shepherd the process during the early years of implementation. A good facilitator helps the organization design and install an effective planning and review process, trains the planning team and the organization in facilitation techniques, intervenes when key organizational or strategic blockages occur, and exits once the team is self-sustaining and self-facilitating.

In nearly all healthcare organizations, the choice of a facilitator is between an internal staff member, typically the director or vice president of planning, and an outside consultant. Occasionally, the facilitator may be an experienced board member, which is generally not recommended, or, in smaller healthcare organizations, the CEO. Once the selection is made, it should be communicated widely in the organization before strategic planning formally commences.

ESTABLISH AND COMMUNICATE THE STRATEGIC PLANNING SCHEDULE

Although strategic planning should be an ongoing activity of every organization, a full strategic plan development process or a complete update of the current plan is usually necessary every three to five years. Most organizations that practice ongoing strategic planning have annual planning cycles and schedules. In such situations, a brief strategic plan update is typically carried out in the first six months of the fiscal year.

Strategic planning experts disagree about the optimal duration of the full strategic planning process. Some believe the plan should be completed as quickly as possible to maintain a high degree of focus. Others believe that an extended schedule allows for broader participation and more creative thinking during the process.

This book endorses a course of action that falls between these two points on the duration spectrum, generally one leaning to the latter view. Here again, senior management must choose from among available alternatives, each with pros and cons. As with the previous steps, the choice should be made deliberately and consciously, before planning activities are initiated, and clearly communicated to all affected constituencies.

ASSEMBLE RELEVANT HISTORICAL DATA

Possessing accurate and relevant data is an asset to strategic planning. Conversely, having inaccurate and incomplete data can be a major impediment to strategic planning. It is never too early to assemble a historical database for strategic planning. Data that profile the past three to five years of the organization's performance and the market in which it operates should be compiled and routinely updated. The specific types of data required and analytical approaches are discussed in Chapter 3. The main point here is twofold:

1. To stress the importance of an early start on the time-consuming data collection process, which is often difficult to complete in a reasonable time frame
2. To emphasize that it is critical to devote ample time and effort to data collection to ensure an accurate and complete database

Discovering at the middle or end of the process that essential data are missing or inaccurate is discouraging at a minimum and disabling at worst, especially if the problem is discovered in a public forum and undermines the credibility of the strategic planning process.

RESOLVE NOT TO OVERANALYZE HISTORICAL DATA

Historical data assembled to aid strategic planning can be a great asset, but data can also trap the organization in a cycle of ineffectiveness. Two major pitfalls hinder effective strategic planning.

Inability to Assemble the Required Database

Determining the amount of historical data required for sound planning is a subjective decision. Often, a few members of a planning team want more or better data and will disable the planning process before it begins or derail it through a series of challenges to its validity.

Undue Focus on Analyses of Past Performance

A related problem is planning team members' penchant for analyzing every facet of historical performance. Determining what analyses are necessary for sound strategic planning will derail efforts to compile superfluous information and limit lengthy delays caused by excessive data gathering.

Although it can be comforting to focus on the past and dwell on the familiar, strategic planning should be oriented toward preparing the organization for the future. Organizations should resolve to use historical data for their intended purpose: guiding future forecasts and strategies.

REVIEW PAST STRATEGIES AND IDENTIFY SUCCESSES AND FAILURES

A review of the organization's past strategies, successes, and failures is often best completed before the strategic planning process starts, for three reasons:

1. It will help determine how best to structure the strategic planning process itself.
2. It will highlight certain types of analyses that may be important to successful planning in a particular situation.
3. It will identify issues the organization's leaders must be aware of as they formulate the new strategies and implementation approaches.

An objective review of past strategies can be enlightening. Often the actual strategies an organization used are different than those proposed in the strategic plan developed for that time frame. Similarly, the actual strategies the organization employed may vary from those that leadership thought were being followed. A review of historical documents by someone outside the inner circle—a new senior staff member or a consultant—and a discussion of what was proposed, was perceived, and actually occurred over the previous three to five years can be a fascinating and important pre–planning process exercise.

As part of this process, what has worked, what has not, and why should be reviewed. Failure to pay adequate attention to unsuccessful strategies in formal planning can lead to recurring mistakes. Thorough, honest evaluation of successful and unsuccessful strategies can help an organization avoid this common pitfall.

CONDUCT STRATEGIC PLANNING ORIENTATION MEETINGS

Orientation meetings set the stage for the official launch of the planning process. Although meetings may be deferred until the strategic planning process formally commences, these meetings should be scheduled and held during the pre-planning stage.

To become fully engaged at the outset of the process, senior management and the strategic planning steering committee might embark on a planning retreat. Here the leadership and committee review the organization's past planning initiatives, including successes and failures; identify and explore important environmental trends and potential impacts; and discuss key planning issues already defined, including potential alternatives to address these issues.

Holding strategic planning orientation sessions for other groups in the organization may be desirable at this point as well. Depending on the size and complexity of the organization and the breadth and depth of participation being sought in the strategic planning process, orientation sessions may be held with the entire board, other members of senior management, physicians, other professional staff, or municipal government leaders or community groups. These sessions usually focus on a few of the areas outlined, such as objectives for strategic planning, the planning process and schedule, or the role of the affected constituencies in the planning process.

PREPARE TO STIMULATE NEW THINKING

Engaging in True Strategic Planning

As the strategic planning process gets under way, the temptation to extrapolate from the performances and experiences of the past and to devise future strategy on this premise must be resisted. In the more orderly and less frenetic world of past decades, good planning strategy may have resulted from this approach. But with changes in the field occurring nonlinearly and at an ever-faster pace, this approach is likely to lead to naive strategies at best and incorrect forecasts and flawed strategic direction at worst.

Avoiding Mimicry

Another problem-laden strategic planning method that healthcare organizations frequently use is adopting or mimicking strategies used by other organizations in demographically similar but more advanced regional markets. This practice often is seen in organizations located in the Midwest or on the East Coast that try to replicate successful methods implemented in California or a similar advanced market. Although this approach may work, it poses significant hazards, including lack of comparability with seemingly similar situations and failure to understand the strategy and plan as it applies to the more advanced market.

While learning can occur in these situations, emphasis should be devoted to breaking new ground and creating a plan that leverages an organization's unique situation and strengths in its market. As is described in chapters 3, 4, and 5, healthcare planners must be thoughtful and creative in accurately characterizing the future environment, understanding implications of changing environmental conditions, and considering potential strategies that enable organizations to achieve strong, beneficial results. Much strategic planning conducted by healthcare organizations assumes a static competitive environment. This approach is at odds with today's reality and will be increasingly so in the more dynamic era of the future.

Stimulating Creative Thinking

With recognition of the importance of strategic thinking in the planning process, this new edition devotes Chapter 11 to stimulating such thinking. What is important to understand at this point is that preparation for the strategic planning process in each organization should include some review of the enormous body of available strategic thinking literature, consideration of organizational needs and potential alternative processes, and selection of techniques that may help the organization leap forward in its strategic development.

REINFORCE FUTURE ORIENTATION

To successfully plan for the future, healthcare organizations must adopt a new perspective on it. This perspective needs to be broader, bolder, and more creative and dynamic than any required in the past. To counter the tendency to overemphasize the past and present circumstances, leaders need to overcompensate and continually push their organizations to break with that past and consider alternative futures that differ vastly from today's known circumstances. Injecting this kind of thinking into healthcare strategic planning invigorates the process and leads to thoughtful plans and strategies that will set the new standard by which successful planning and development are measured in the twenty-first century.

CONCLUSION

Before initiating the strategic planning process, organizations may find it helpful to review some requirements for effective planning.

Exhibit 2.1: Requirements for Effective Planning

Community Support	Leadership	Direction	Resources	Structure	Timing	*What you feel:*
	✓	✓	✓	✓	✓	Frustration
✓		✓	✓	✓	✓	Confusion
✓	✓		✓	✓	✓	Fibrillation
✓	✓	✓		✓	✓	Stagnation
✓	✓	✓	✓		✓	Uselessness
✓	✓	✓	✓	✓		Irrelevance

© 2011 Health Strategies & Solutions, Inc.

Exhibit 2.1 presents a useful starting point for discussion. If strategic planning is to be judged successful, especially in nonprofit organizations, it must have all the elements identified in the column headings. Lacking even one element will lead to the problems described in the rows of the exhibit, and, ultimately, failure to plan effectively for the future.

Even 30 years after its emergence, healthcare strategic planning remains a relatively immature practice despite its growing sophistication. Within this chapter alone, healthcare strategic planning has been characterized as historically focused rather than future oriented, lacking creativity, preoccupied with mimicry, haphazardly applied, and poorly planned for. One part of the problem is a lack of drive toward clear, compelling results; another part is a failure to adequately *prepare to* plan by staff and other important members of the organization. This chapter addresses both of these deficits and, it is hoped, heightens awareness of the need to prepare for successful strategic planning.

CHAPTER 3

Activity I: Analyzing the Environment

To prophesy is extremely difficult . . . especially with respect
to the future.

—*Chinese proverb*

When it comes to the future, there are three kinds of people:
those who let it happen, those who make it happen, and
those who wonder what happened.

—*John M. Richardson Jr.*

LOOKING FORWARD VERSUS LOOKING BACKWARD

Strategic planning typically begins with an analysis of the current situation and recent history of the organization referred to as the situation analysis or environmental assessment (see Exhibit 3.1).

The environmental assessment should

- identify past successes and failures: what has worked, what has not, and why;
- give trustees and others less knowledgeable about the organization a solid grounding for constructive involvement;

Exhibit 3.1: Developing the Plan: Environmental Assessment

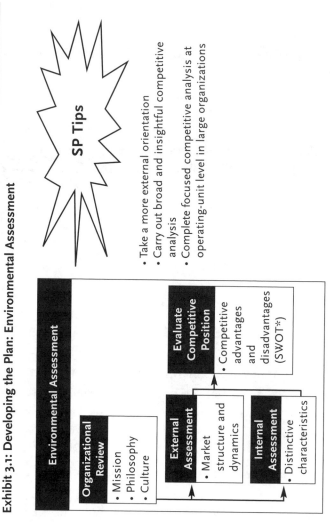

SP Tips

- Take a more external orientation
- Carry out broad and insightful competitive analysis
- Complete focused competitive analysis at operating-unit level in large organizations

Environmental Assessment

Organizational Review
- Mission
- Philosophy
- Culture

External Assessment
- Market structure and dynamics

Internal Assessment
- Distinctive characteristics

Evaluate Competitive Position
- Competitive advantages and disadvantages (SWOT*)

* SWOT = strengths, weaknesses, opportunities, and threats.

© 2011 Health Strategies & Solutions, Inc.

- help determine what factors are subject to the organization's control and influence; and
- identify how external forces might affect the organization in the future.

Although the environmental assessment may be viewed as mere busywork for the planning staff before real strategic planning begins, it has valid and important purposes that should be enumerated and highlighted at the start of the assessment. Among them, as the first activity in the planning process, the environmental assessment largely sets the tone for the strategic plan and is an indicator for how the rest of the planning process is likely to unfold by examining the following questions:

- Will the process be comprehensive in scope?
- Will it involve key organizational stakeholders in a constructive way?
- Will it be highly structured or loosely organized?
- Have the outcomes of the strategic planning process been clearly articulated, and will this process drive toward their achievement?
- Is a planning schedule being followed, and will that planning lead to action?

As discussed in Chapter 2, many planning efforts get off to a poor start because the planning process and activities lack sufficient advance conceptualization, organization, or explanation to the whole organization. The environmental assessment, if poorly planned and executed, can derail subsequent strategic planning activities. For example, the staff may become enmeshed in data gathering and analysis, bogging down the entire planning process early—a problem known as analysis paralysis. Guidelines and

Exhibit 3.2: Minimum Data Requirements for the Environmental Assessment

Internal	External
• Characteristics and utilization of major programs and services • Key indicators: facilities, equipment, and staff • Financial performance and position	• Major demographic and economic indicators • Major technology, reimbursement, and regulatory factors • Position of major programs and services • Profile and analysis of key competitors • Future market size and characteristics

© 2011 Health Strategies & Solutions, Inc.

Exhibit 3.3: Online Healthcare Data Resources

• National Center for Health Statistics	www.cdc.gov/nchs
• Agency for Healthcare Research and Quality	www.ahrq.gov
• Centers for Medicare & Medicaid Services	www.cms.hhs.gov
• Centers for Disease Control and Prevention	www.cdc.gov
• Health Resources and Services Administration	www.hrsa.gov
• National Cancer Institute	www.cancer.gov
• American Hospital Association	www.aha.org
• American Medical Association	www.ama-assn.org
• The Dartmouth Atlas of Health Care	www.dartmouthatlas.org
• State-specific hospital discharge databases	

Exhibit 3.4: Creative Data Gathering for the Environmental Assessment: Competitor Intelligence

Hard Data	Soft Data
• State licensure and other state filings • 990 and 10-K reports and other federal filings • Hospital associations • Public vendors	• Annual reports • Web sites • Public relations releases or brochures • Newspaper articles • Speeches by executives • Former employees

© 2011 Health Strategies & Solutions, Inc.

resources for effectively carrying out data gathering—a complicated and controversial task—are provided in exhibits 3.2, 3.3, and 3.4.

While it is important to compile a database that clearly reflects the organization's historical performance and market, strategic planning is not primarily an exercise in plotting historical patterns and then extrapolating. Reviewing recent history and analyzing successes and failures is a comforting activity. But little is gained from overanalysis of the past, and whatever momentum and excitement the organization may be able to create at the initiation of strategic planning will likely be lost if historical performance becomes the major focus of the strategic planning process.

This chapter examines the two components of the environmental assessment—the internal and external assessments—and the main outputs they should produce to facilitate the remaining activities of the strategic planning process.

APPROACH TO THE INTERNAL ASSESSMENT

The internal assessment combines data analysis with qualitative information and analysis to formulate an accurate profile of the historical performance of the organization. Along with the external assessment, discussed in the next section, it establishes the organization's strengths, weaknesses, opportunities, and threats (SWOT) and identifies competitive advantages and disadvantages (discussed later) that serve as a springboard to subsequent strategic planning activities. The internal assessment has five main components.

1. Review Role Statements and Organizational Framework

The first component of the internal assessment is a high-level review that determines whether the organization does as it says it will do in terms of its mission, vision, and values statements and whether its structure and processes allow it to achieve its purpose and business aims. The review includes an assessment of its current statements (mission, vision, values) and a comparison of these to recent performance. An assessment of program development and financial performance is also carried out. The structures of governance and management are evaluated in light of the mission, vision, and values assessments and in comparison to similar organizations; a review of their effectiveness, on the basis of internal information and industry norms where available, completes this task.

2. Analyze Characteristics and Utilization Trends

All the programs and services of an organization should be inventoried in the trends analysis task. The top 75 to 80 percent (as measured by volume or financial contribution) should have a profile that includes capacity, volumes, and key resource attributes for the past three to five years. Profiling low-volume programs and services or those that perform poorly financially may also be worthwhile as a prelude to considering downsizing or divestiture.

3. Conduct Primary Market Research

Market research has two primary purposes: (1) to gather pertinent information on the strengths and weaknesses of the organization and its competitors in the marketplace and (2) to involve organization leadership constructively and broadly early in the strategic planning process. This task should begin with a review of any recent (within the past one to three years) primary market research. Then, additional research can be initiated, including personal interviews, focus groups, online or written surveys, and telephone surveys.

Internal research targets typically include board members, physicians, other health professionals, and upper and middle management staff; in some cases, all employees may be research targets. Market research, when performed well, provides almost limitless returns. Although the substantive value of the market research may diminish significantly as greater amounts of research are carried out, the political value of soliciting and carefully listening to organizational leaders' and stakeholders' opinions should not be ignored. Researchers must clearly indicate that they are listening through note taking at the outset, and through feedback following the research.

4. Analyze Other Critical Resources

Resource analysis generally focuses on facilities, equipment, and staff to identify major assets and liabilities. Comparison to industry norms and competitors is appropriate.

5. Analyze Financial Performance and Position

The past three to five years of financial performance for the organization and its major components should be profiled and compared to industry norms and competitors. If the organization has already prepared future financial projections for the next three to five years, these should be included in the analysis.

The Internal Assessment's End Product

The product of the internal assessment should be a summary of the results that contains a maximum of ten charts or tables, with modest narration or highlighting of key points. (The largest and most complex healthcare organizations may need more than ten exhibits, but not many more.) While three to five times as many analytical tables and other supporting documents may be prepared and available as backup, the internal assessment summary should be brief for ease of understanding and use.

APPROACH TO THE EXTERNAL ASSESSMENT

The external assessment, like the internal assessment, should be an accurate profile of the organization's historical performance as it relates to the marketplace in which it operates. The external assessment profiles the historical performance and evolution of the marketplace and initiates the process of looking forward by explicitly considering market trends and forecasts. The external assessment has five main components.

1. Review Demographic, Economic, and Health Status Conditions

This task identifies the broadest trends and variables that have had and will have an impact on organizational performance. While key community demographic, economic, and health status indicators for the past three to five years should be profiled and forecasts provided for the next five to ten years, if available, it is important to

Exhibit 3.5: Major Dynamics in North American Children's Hospitals, 2009

- Rising costs of care
- Use of technology
- Meeting even higher philanthropic demands
- Higher acuity patients
- Managing children (and young adults) with chronic diseases
- Pediatric subspecialty shortages
- Geographic distribution of services
- Capacity constraints
- Academic pressures
- Demonstrating quality
- Increasingly informed healthcare consumers

Source: BC Children's Hospital (2009). Used with permission.

note that minor shifts in these measures are of minimal or no consequence to the strategic planning process. Organizations should take care not to overreach and instead should aim to complete a review with a scope that is general and high level rather than detailed. In addition to identifying broad trends, this analysis is occasionally useful in identifying geographical areas or population segments with strong potential for future cultivation.

2. Review the State of Healthcare Delivery

The purpose of reviewing applicable healthcare technology, delivery, reimbursement, regulatory, teaching, and research trends is to identify any major environmental (largely state or national) influences that have affected and may affect the organization's performance. (An example of such a review for a children's hospital is shown in Exhibit 3.5.) Major trends in each category should be profiled for the past three to five years. Forecasts, including potential alternative scenarios, for the next three to five years should be identified and discussed.

With predictions that reimbursement constraints will continue to dramatically affect hospitals and systems, this issue deserves particular attention going forward. Technological and pharmaceutical advances should also be considered among the major environmental influences in the future.

3. Analyze Competitors

Analyzing competitors is the most important task—and often the most difficult one—to complete well in the environmental assessment, so substantial effort should be assigned to it. Competitor data in healthcare can be incomplete and out of date, although, increasingly, good information can be collected with some hard work and resourcefulness.

Competitors may operate on a variety of levels. Some organizations may compete in most or all service categories, whereas others may do so in one or a few select niches. Competitor data should be collected from local, regional, state, and national sources such as HealthGrades, the Joint Commission Quality Check, payer provider directories, bond rating agencies, the American Hospital Directory, AHA Hospital Statistics, provider websites, and business journals and newspapers.

Because of this topic's importance and evidence that many healthcare organizations have historically failed to complete this task adequately, a three-part example from a strategic plan (exhibits 3.6, 3.7, and 3.8) demonstrates a rigorous analysis.

4. Conduct Primary Market Research

The market research task in conducting an external assessment parallels that of the internal assessment but focuses on parties external to the organization. The purpose of market research is to gather pertinent information on the organization's position in its mar-

Exhibit 3.6: Analysis of XYZ's Competitors' Strategies, 2009

Strategy	System A	System B	AMC A	AMC B	System C	Specialty Hospital
Quality position	✪	●	●	●	○	✪
Market share	✪	●	✪	✪	○	●
Marketing and consumer preference	○	●	●	●	○	✪
Facilities	○	●	✪	✪	○	○
GME/research	○	○	●	●	○	○
Partnerships	✪	●	●	●	○	○

Symbol	Description
●	High risk to XYZ
✪	Moderate risk to XYZ
○	Low risk to XYZ

© 2011 Health Strategies & Solutions, Inc.

ketplace relative to its competitors and likely changes in key external factors. Recent (within the past one to three years) primary market research should be reviewed before proceeding with this task. Appropriate research may include personal interviews, focus groups, online or written surveys, and telephone surveys. Research targets in the external assessment typically include competitor organizations' senior management, other people knowledgeable about the healthcare delivery system, and community leaders.

5. Assess Market Forecasts and Implications

Population changes, economic indicators, and healthcare delivery-specific parameters for the community that have already have been compiled in publicly available forecasts—should be obtained and assessed. If forecasts need to be prepared, at a minimum, projections should use appropriate forecasting techniques for major

Exhibit 3.7: XYZ's Future Competitive Environment and Planning Implications, 2013

Strategy	System A	System B	System C	Specialty Hospital	AMC A	AMC B	Physician Groups	Planning Implications for XYZ
Development of COEs, specialty care	X	X			X	X		Enhance programs based on quality, other differentiating factors
Growth in ambulatory care	X				X	X	X	Enhance/develop suburban outposts
Aggressive pursuit of suburban market	X				X	X	X	Strengthen referral relationships
Survival mode			X	X				Consider candidates for affliation or merger/ acquisition

Competitors are moving forward very aggressively, raising the cost and difficulty of competitive success for XYZ

Notes: Physician groups were not significant competition in 2009, so they are not included in Exhibit 3.6

COE = center of excellence

© 2011 Health Strategies & Solutions, Inc.

Exhibit 3.8: Potential Future Competitor Positioning Re: XYZ, 2010–2013

Organization	Baseline Forecast	Aggressive Forecast (in addition to baseline)	Declining Forecast
System A	• Builds new hospital • Continues to migrate toward tertiary services • Strengthens ties with private physicians • Leverages existing partnerships	• Breakthrough in service mix (e.g., cardiac surgery) • Major academic affiliation • National prominence for IT or other innovations	• Becomes overextended and pulls back on investments and programs
System B	• Draws more local referrals and basic ED activity • Creates new partnerships with physician groups	• Infuses major resources through system connections	• Financial erosion to a safety-net hospital
Physician Groups	• Consolidation of small groups • Stronger ties to health systems • Office-based ancillaries	• Larger groups develop major ambulatory care facilities	• Regulation forces physician groups out of ancillary business
Etc.	Etc.	Etc.	Etc.

health service components, including acute, post-acute, and ambulatory care services by major service lines.

The External Assessment's End Product

A summary of the market structure and dynamics should be prepared in parallel form to that of the internal assessment. A brief report with no more than ten charts and tables accompanied by modest narration or highlighting of key points should suffice. Additional materials may be available for back-up support if needed.

KEY OUTPUTS OF THE INTERNAL AND EXTERNAL ASSESSMENTS

The internal and external assessments need to produce three main outputs for subsequent activities: (1) a succinct, pointed, and honest statement of the organization's competitive advantages and disadvantages in the marketplace; (2) assumptions about the future environment; and (3) considering the content of the first two outputs, an appraisal of key planning issues that require resolution in the strategic planning process.

Competitive Advantages and Disadvantages

No particular approach or format for determining and displaying competitive advantages and disadvantages is universally accepted. In general, the two most reliable measures of competitive advantage or disadvantage are market share and bond rating. Upward historical trends in these variables usually indicate a strong competitive position. However, trends seen in healthcare organizations are rarely clear cut. Simply focusing on bond rating and market share may, for example, mask major shifts in competitive position due to the lagged effect of capital or human investments.

Commonly used formats for displaying competitive advantage and disadvantage are (1) a SWOT summary and (2) a straightforward enumeration of competitive advantages and disadvantages. Examples of the typical outputs of each are shown in exhibits 3.9 and 3.10.

While a lengthy listing of SWOT or competitive advantages and disadvantages may initially be generated, the final list should be refined to a one-page summary. As the exhibits show, items may

Exhibit 3.9: Small Rural System Strategic Profile

Strengths	Weaknesses
• Excellent financials (particularly for hospital and home care agency) • Relatively large, subspecialized, high-quality medical staff • Home care has very high market share and recent growth • Quality at hospital and home care agency • Broad range of services • Community support and fundraising • Geographic isolation	• Nursing home facilities • Organizational structure cumbersome • Hospital site constrained • Hospital vulnerable at periphery of service area • Somewhat parochial and resistant to change • Information systems • Market share in surgical services and medical subspecialties

Opportunities	Threats
• Addition of more physicians to medical staff especially in key specialties and primary care at periphery • Senior services • Further penetration into southern part of region • New service development • Acquisition of other local nursing home and rationalization of nursing home services	• Potential demise of protective state regulation • Further reach of two nearby large hospitals and metro area providers into region • Further reimbursement cutbacks • Competition from physicians for outpatient ancillaries

Exhibit 3.10: Large Rural Healthcare System Competitive Analysis

Competitive Advantages	Competitive Disadvantages
• Dominant provider in a 15-county region • Strong financial performance and position • Market share growing • Viewed as the quality provider • Competitive costs and prices	• Complacent • Large, cumbersome, and bureaucratic • Losing share at periphery of region • Strong competitors outside the region are moving in

be drawn from any category of the internal and external assessments, but not every assessment category needs to be represented in the final summary.

The purpose of the advantages/disadvantages analysis is to provide organizational leadership with a clear assessment of where the organization stands in its competitive marketplace. Little benefit is derived from applying overly complicated analysis to achieve the results. Leadership must use its skills, experience, and judgment to synthesize all of the external assessment findings and determine the organization's real advantages and disadvantages.

Assumptions About the Future

Up to this point in its process, the environmental assessment has been concerned primarily with the past. The remainder of the assessment and the strategic planning process shifts the focus to the future.

The first forward-looking task is to develop a picture of the future environment, at least three to five years hence and perhaps further, in which the organization will operate. This forecast should consider key external factors (some local or regional, others state or national) that may have a significant impact on the organization's future strategies. It should not be strictly numerical, for example, delineating market size and the precise level of reimbursement changes, but rather a qualitative and macro-level view of significant future and external influences.

The predictions of healthcare futurists and the forecasts from publications and associations that track emerging trends can help healthcare organizations formulate their own assumptions (see the suggested readings at the end of this chapter for examples of available resources). Hamel and Prahalad (1994) write that few organizations spend an adequate amount of time thinking about the future, noting that "senior managers devote less than 3% . . . of their time to building a *corporate* perspective on the future. In some companies, the figure is less than 1%. Our experience suggests that to develop a distinctive point of view about the future, senior managers must be willing to devote considerably more of their time" (emphasis in original).

Historically, healthcare organizations and the general business community have predicated much of their planning on one view of the future environment—usually a linear extrapolation of the past—rather than evaluating a wide range of possible futures. The upheavals in healthcare and other fields illustrate how this singular view of the future has led to major errors in organization strategy and legitimate concern about the wisdom of planning for the future within a limited environmental context.

In the 1970s General Motors failed to explore fully the impact of the Organization of the Petroleum Exporting Countries (OPEC) on globalization, environmentalism, and the importance of quality and speed in manufacturing (Schoemaker 1995). In the 1980s, IBM and Digital Equipment Corp. failed to account for the consequences of personal computers (Schoemaker 1995). According to Hamel and Prahalad (1994), "If senior executives don't have reasonably detailed answers to the 'future' questions, and if the answers they have are not significantly different from the 'today' answers, there is little chance that their companies will remain market leaders."

Planning for the future within a narrow, limited environmental context may have been acceptable in the more static, highly regulated healthcare environment that prevailed through the early 1990s. However, this approach is no longer feasible and constitutes one of the main differences between contemporary strategic planning methods and those of even the recent past.

To ensure that a broader perspective is adopted, alternative futures should be defined and discussed fully. Products of the environmental assessment may need to be revised or fine-tuned after completing this task.

Many excellent references offer approaches for developing alternative future scenarios. Among these, Schoemaker (1995) recommends the following steps in scenario development:

1. Define the scope (time frame and scope of analysis)
2. Identify the major stakeholders
3. Identify basic trends
4. Identify key uncertainties
5. Construct initial scenario themes
6. Check for consistency and plausibility
7. Develop preliminary scenarios
8. Identify additional research needs
9. Develop quantitative models, as applicable
10. Evolve toward a final scenario (iteratively, converge toward the scenario that will be used)

This approach enables organizational leadership to consider and seriously analyze diverse alternative futures and distill a composite scenario from this broad view of the future. In contrast, most healthcare organizations typically rely—explicitly or implicitly—on the planning staff to develop a single future environmental scenario by extrapolating current trends and incorporating current hot issues.

Exhibit 3.11: Future Assumptions Regarding the National and Local Market: FY2010 to FY2015

- Provider success will be based on demonstrated quality outcomes and customer service.
- Economic difficulties in the United States and local area will directly affect the healthcare economy.
- There is a greater potential for national and/or state healthcare reform.
- Financial pressures will be exacerbated due to commercial payment increases slowing to single-digit levels, state budget issues, and a large number of uninsured individuals in the state (in the absence of major healthcare reform).
- There is an increased likelihood of hospital closures due to poor financial performance, and industry consolidation will occur, too.
- An increasing proportion of physicians will be employed by hospitals or systems.
- Technological advances will continue to shift services to the outpatient setting.
- Medical manpower shortages and competition for labor will increase.

© 2011 Health Strategies & Solutions, Inc.

Regardless of the approach used, the result should be an explicit set of underlying assumptions about the future, on which the remaining planning analyses and outputs will be based. Exhibit 3.11 presents an example of the results of this process.

As the example illustrates, the assumptions should be stated briefly to avoid unnecessarily complicating the presentation of the future environment in which the organization will operate. This concise, simple summary of a potential future environment is a powerful guide by which to consider, or in many cases reconsider, critical planning issues and, subsequently, organizational mission and vision.

Identification of Planning Issues

The final task in the environmental assessment is to determine what critical planning issues need to be resolved during the strategic planning process. All of the preceding analysis feeds into this

Exhibit 3.12: Results of Environmental Assessment: Framework for Critical Issues Facing Healthcare Organizations

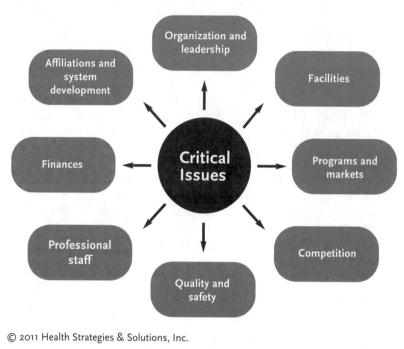

final result. The determination is subjective and usually evolves through an iterative process of some or all of the steps described in the next paragraph, depending on the size and complexity of the organization, the issues it faces, and the extent to which participative processes are used in strategic planning.

After the planning analyst or planning staff select an initial list of issues, senior management team members review and revise the list, alone or together. The list may then go to the strategic planning committee members, individually or collectively, who will perform the same review. The issue listing may then be accepted as a basis for moving forward or returned to the planning or senior management staff for further work.

Exhibit 3.12 shows a framework for categorizing the types of critical planning issues that emerge. Typical critical planning issues that are common to strategic plans today are

Exhibit 3.13: Where is BC Children's Now? Key Strategic Planning Issues, 2009

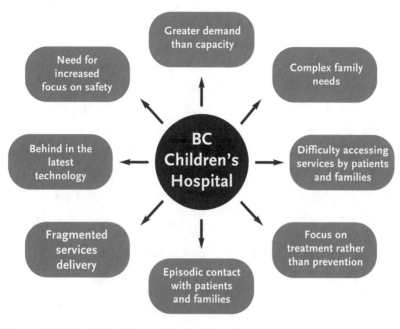

Source: BC Children's Hospital, 2009. Used with permission.

- developing clinical programs and improving competitive positioning,
- strengthening financial performance,
- demonstrating value,
- building mutually beneficial relationships with the medical staff, and
- constructing an effective delivery system.

Exhibit 3.13 shows an interesting and thoughtful example of critical issues identified in the strategic plan of a Canadian children's hospital.

A variety of largely operational and quasi-strategic matters frequently emerge as critical issues in the environmental assessment. Leaders are often tempted to enumerate dozens of "important" issues that need to be resolved to ensure future success. But by

Exhibit 3.14: One Healthcare System's Critical Issues Categorization

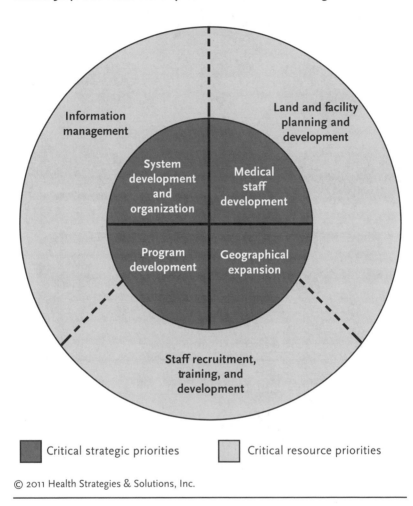

© 2011 Health Strategies & Solutions, Inc.

doing so, they sacrifice strategic clarity and precision in the name of comprehensiveness and political expediency.

Only a limited number of issues can and should be dealt with in the strategic planning process if the planning is to lead to a successful outcome. Exhibit 3.14 depicts how one healthcare delivery system subdivided the defined issues into two categories: critical strategic priorities and critical resource priorities. This approach is one reasonable way to handle an otherwise thorny political situation.

Few healthcare organizations have so many critical issues that they cannot be condensed to five to ten strategic issue categories. Failure to produce a limited number of issues to address in subsequent planning activities almost always dooms the strategic planning process. It is impossible to effectively tackle an excessive number of issues concurrently and may confuse organizational leadership about what issues are truly critical to strategic development.

CONCLUSION

A brief and high-level list of planning issues that require resolution is an excellent springboard to the next two planning activities: establishing overall or corporate direction and formulating core strategies. Such a list reduces voluminous data and other information collected during the environmental assessment to a manageable amount and energizes organizational leadership to move forward on strategic planning with a clear focus on issues of immense importance to the organization.

SUGGESTED READINGS TO TRACK EMERGING HEALTHCARE TRENDS

American Hospital Association. "AHA Environmental Scan." Published annually in the September issue of *H&HN*. www.hhnmag.com/hhnmag_app/jsp/articledisplay.jsp?domain=HHNMAG&dcrpath=HHNMAG/Article/data/09SEP2011/0911HHN_Feature_Gatefold

American Hospital Association Resource Center. Blog. http://aharesourcecenter.wordpress.com/

Health Affairs. Published monthly. www.healthaffairs.org/

"Healthcare Business and Policy Outlook." *Modern Healthcare*, published annually in the first issue of the year for this magazine. www.modernhealthcare.com/

Healthcare Financial Management. Published monthly. www.hfma.org/hfm/

Journal of Healthcare Management. Published bimonthly. www.ache.org/pubs/jhmsub.cfm

Medicare Payment Advisory Commission. Report to the Congress: Medicare Payment Policy. Published annually in March. www.medpac.gov/

Society for Healthcare Strategy & Market Development and Health Administration Press. *Futurescan: Healthcare Trends and Implications.* Published annually.

"The State of Medical Practice." *MGMA Connexion.* Published annually in the January issue of this magazine.

CHAPTER 4

Activity II: Identifying Organizational Direction

No wind favors the ship that has no charted course.

—*Nautical saying*

Good business leaders create a vision, articulate the vision, passionately own the vision, and relentlessly drive it to completion.

—*Jack Welch*

The second activity of the strategic planning process, identifying organizational direction, initiates in earnest the process of looking forward to chart what the organization's future might be. This activity sets high-level direction encompassing mission, vision, overall organizational strategy, and values. Subsequent activities address important components of future direction and the particular aspects of implementation. Exhibit 4.1 provides a context for the principal outputs of the organizational direction activity.

REVIEW OF THE LITERATURE

The strategic planning literature highlights the importance of a clear mission and vision to the organization's future success.

Exhibit 4.1: Organizational Direction

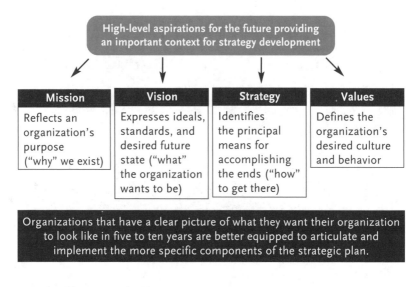

High-level aspirations for the future providing an important context for strategy development

Mission	Vision	Strategy	Values
Reflects an organization's purpose ("why" we exist)	Expresses ideals, standards, and desired future state ("what" the organization wants to be)	Identifies the principal means for accomplishing the ends ("how" to get there)	Defines the organization's desired culture and behavior

Organizations that have a clear picture of what they want their organization to look like in five to ten years are better equipped to articulate and implement the more specific components of the strategic plan.

© 2011 Health Strategies & Solutions, Inc.

Swayne, Duncan, and Ginter (2008) note that mission, vision, values, and strategic goals are accurately called directional strategies because they guide strategists in making key organizational decisions. Coile (1994) describes the interrelationship between vision and strategy as an arrow-to-target process. A shared vision is the target, and strategic planning is the arrow. Clark (2011) writes that organizational vision has three operational functions: a cognitive function to educate, an emotional function to motivate, and an organizational function to coordinate. When all three functions are in place and actively applied, the vision guides the answers to thousands of operational questions and leads to coordinated, effective, and efficient action (Clark 2011).

There are, however, caveats to developing mission and vision statements. Bart (2002) writes, "For many senior executives, mission statements don't seem to be worth the paper on which they are written. They don't seem to be of any value." Nonetheless, he goes on to say, "Surprisingly, mission statements (and their accompanying vision and values proclamations) continue to be considered one of the most popular management tools in the world and have even been ranked at least in the top two practices in global usage by Bain & Company since 1993."

As Bart (2002) suggests and as this author's experience validates, the reason for the popularity and prevalence of mission and vision statements is that they make a promise and focus the organization's activities on fulfilling it. Most often, healthcare organizations that clearly express their basic purpose in a mission statement and paint an accurate picture of what they want their organization to look like in five to ten years in a vision statement stand a good chance of articulating and implementing the specific components of the strategic plan, thereby realizing that vision. Failure to specify a mission that is compelling and unique to the healthcare organization, or to define a clear and exciting vision, hinders attempts to resolve strategic issues and to make progress toward a better future.

Kaplan, Norton, and Barrows (2008) note that if vision statements are to guide strategy development, they must be inspirational, aspirational, and measurable. To be useful, a statement should also provide a clear focus for the strategy by including a measurable outcome and a distinct target. Kaplan, Norton, and Barrows suggest that a well-crafted vision statement should include three components: a quantified success indicator, a definition of a niche, and a timeline. These three components are evident in the example from Leeds University in the United Kingdom (Kaplan, Norton, and Barrows 2008):

> By 2015 (*timeline*), our distinctive ability to integrate world-class research, scholarship, and education (*niche*) will have secured us a place among the top 50 universities in the world (*quantifiable success indicator*).

Finally, Porter (1996) cautions that all too frequently in US industry, "Bit by bit, almost imperceptibly, management tools have taken the place of strategy. As managers push to improve on all fronts, they move farther away from viable competitive positions." By failing to focus on what will distinguish their organizations in the future, and thus on the essence of effective organizational direction, these companies have difficulty translating gains in operational improvements into sustained profitability.

GUIDELINES FOR DEVELOPING AN EFFECTIVE ORGANIZATIONAL DIRECTION

While specifying direction is necessary and important, developing effective organizational direction statements is a monumental challenge, especially in healthcare organizations. Common problems in direction statements are extreme wordiness; confusion of mission, vision, strategy, and values and a mixture of some in each statement; redundancy among statements; lack of precision; and failure to be farsighted.

Effective statements must be, above all, meaningful, motivational, and memorable. For example, The Joint Commission expects the rank-and-file employees (and especially the leadership) in the organizations it reviews to know their mission statements.

How many mission statements are clear and succinct enough that the organization's employees can readily restate it?

Exhibit 4.2 provides a summary of the guidelines for successfully navigating this activity of the strategic planning process. Key points include the following:

- **Sharp, tailored, directional statements are produced.** These statements should be highly focused and specific to the particular organization that created them; platitudes and verbosity have no place here.
- **For any complex, multi-entity organization, one vision and one direction are essential.** All subsidiaries must move in the same direction; major, and sometimes minor, differences in vision and direction are divisive and potentially destructive.

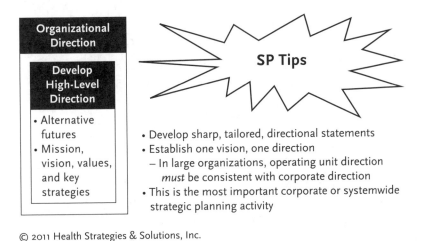

Exhibit 4.2: Developing the Plan: Organizational Direction

Organizational Direction

Develop High-Level Direction

- Alternative futures
- Mission, vision, values, and key strategies

SP Tips

- Develop sharp, tailored, directional statements
- Establish one vision, one direction
  - In large organizations, operating unit direction *must* be consistent with corporate direction
- This is the most important corporate or systemwide strategic planning activity

© 2011 Health Strategies & Solutions, Inc.

- **Organizational direction is the most critical part of the board's and CEO's contribution to strategic planning.** It must emanate from and be fully supported by all elements of corporate or system leadership.

If planning for the future position of the organization starts with a poorly conceived, uncertain, or confusing directional statement, the planning process may eventually derail and it will be difficult, if not impossible, to get it back on track. Beginning with clear organizational direction, on the other hand, helps focus the subsequent, detailed strategy formulation and implementation planning activities, making it critical to strategic planning success. The following sections discuss development of the mission statement, the vision statement, the overall strategy, and the values statement.

DEVELOPMENT OF THE MISSION STATEMENT

Mission statements should be relatively timeless in the absence of significant organizational change. Some organizations' current statements will not require alterations as part of the strategic plan development process. If reexamination and retooling of the mission statement are called for, the starting point should be the current statement. Most mission statements created by healthcare organizations in recent years have two main problems. First, they are lengthy and cumbersome, and second, mission is often confused with strategy.

Mission Statement Characteristics

Effective mission statements are brief and fundamental statements of organizational purpose. A mission statement should clearly communicate to the board, employees, and other internal and external constituencies why the organization exists and what important purpose it intends to achieve. To accomplish this end, the mission statement must be short and to the point. Many experts believe that the most effective mission statements are one sentence in length at most. Influential management consultant, writer, and professor Peter Drucker said that the content of a mission statement should be small enough to fit on a T-shirt (Drucker 1998).

Several examples of recently developed mission statements for healthcare organizations, as well as examples from major companies outside the healthcare field, are presented in Exhibit 4.3. Note the precision, clarity, and brevity of the non-healthcare mission statements compared with even these exceptional examples of healthcare mission statements. Interesting, too, is how 3M and Nike capture the essence of their purpose without resorting to descriptions of the business, products, or markets. These statements should inspire healthcare leaders to think carefully and creatively about the true purpose of their organizations.

Mission Statement Development Process

The mission statement development process varies by organization, but most include significant input from the board, as this

Exhibit 4.3: Mission Statement Examples

Non-healthcare
3M: To solve unsolved problems innovatively
Nike: To bring inspiration and innovation to every athlete in the world
Google: To organize the world's information and make it universally accessible and useful

Healthcare
Barnes-Jewish Hospital (St. Louis, Missouri): We take exceptional care of people. • By providing world-class healthcare • By delivering care in a compassionate, respectful and responsive way • By advancing medical knowledge and continuously improving our practices • By educating current and future generations of healthcare professionals
Hunterdon Healthcare System (Flemington, New Jersey): Hunterdon Healthcare System exists to prevent and treat disease, illness, and injury, to seek cures, to relieve pain, to give comfort, and to inspire a healthy way of living.
Sentara Healthcare (Norfolk, Virginia): We improve health every day.

involvement is the board's most fundamental contribution to organization policy and strategic direction. Development begins with the strategic planning committee, which may hold two to three sessions at least partly devoted to a discussion of mission. These sessions typically encompass

- scenario development and generation of a composite future scenario (as discussed in Chapter 3),
- review of the definition of a mission statement and examination of the current statement,
- review of other healthcare organizations' mission statements (and possibly some non-healthcare mission statements), and
- review and modification of a new draft mission statement.

Strategic planning committee or board members should not be wordsmiths for the proposed mission statement. They should instead concentrate on what the mission statement is trying to convey, focusing on substantive changes in content. A group discussion is not the place to rewrite, in whole or in part, the mission statement, as it is a cumbersome, tedious, and ultimately unproductive approach. Drafting or redrafting the document should be left to an individual or a small group once the discussion sessions have yielded the statement's focus.

DEVELOPMENT OF THE VISION STATEMENT

Vision statements and mission statements are usually developed simultaneously and follow the same process and general principles. The distinction between mission statements and vision statements is that mission statements are not time limited whereas vision statements refer to a particular future point or period and generally must be updated and revised with each complete strategic planning process.

Vision Statement Characteristics

Unlike the mission statement, the current vision statement will likely require substantial change if it is to be an effective guide for the organization's future direction. But many current vision statements share two main problems with mission statements—cumbersome length and inappropriate inclusion of strategy.

Effective vision statements conform to the guidelines listed in Exhibit 4.1. The vision statement should be a vehicle by which to communicate to internal constituencies a preferred future state of the organization, usually as long as ten years out. It should be a challenge given current circumstances and conditions, and it should represent such an exciting and desirable state of being that it motivates and energizes all elements of the organization to achieve that state through the detailed strategies and actions that support it. The vision statement should project far enough that the future is unpredictable. The time frame should encourage organizational leaders to be imaginative in their views of the future characteristics of the organization while avoiding the urge to analyze their way into the future. Kouzes and Posner (2002) suggest, "Effective visions possess four important attributes: idealism, uniqueness, future orientation, and imagery."

Several examples of healthcare organization vision statements that conform to this description are presented in Exhibit 4.4, along with a few classic examples from major corporations outside the healthcare field.

Here, as with the mission statement examples, the precision, clarity, and brevity of the non-healthcare examples are striking. Those examples also illustrate the recommended vision principles—stretching, motivating, and inspiring the organizations to achieve what nearly all experts would have deemed improbable, if not impossible, at the time they were developed. Healthcare organizations are making progress in vision development, and the examples in Exhibit 4.4 illustrate this effort.

An example that may provide additional insights into organizational vision is the vision statement in the 2008 strategic plan of Our Health System (name changed to disguise the organization's identity). Our Health System aspires to be in the top tier of medical centers nationally but recognizes that this vision could be a 20-year journey (see Exhibit 4.5). Our Health System has set its long-range vision and has also established interim five-year targets as part of its recent strategic planning efforts.

Vision Statement Development Process

The suggestions discussed earlier related to the mission statement apply in this task, too. Interactions among the board, strategic plan-

Exhibit 4.4: Vision Statement Examples

Non-healthcare
Ford (early 1900s): Democratize the automobile
Sony (early 1950s): Become the company most known for changing the worldwide poor-quality image of Japanese products
Stanford University (1940s): Become the Harvard of the West
Healthcare
Barnes-Jewish Hospital (St. Louis, Missouri): BJH will be the best teaching hospital in the world, coupling unparalleled clinical expertise with a new standard in health care for compassion and service.
Along with our partner, Washington University School of Medicine, [we] will be the best academic medical center in the country recognized for excellence in research, teaching, and quality and safety of patient care.
Hunterdon Healthcare System: It is the vision of Hunterdon Healthcare System that all individuals within its healthcare reach be connected to its services and an active partner in its mission.
Sentara: To be the healthcare choice of the communities we serve.

Exhibit 4.5: Road Map to Achieve Our Health System's Long-Range Vision

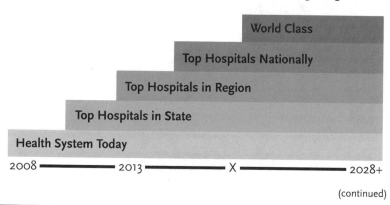

(continued)

Exhibit 4.5: Road Map to Achieve Our Health System's Long-Range Vision

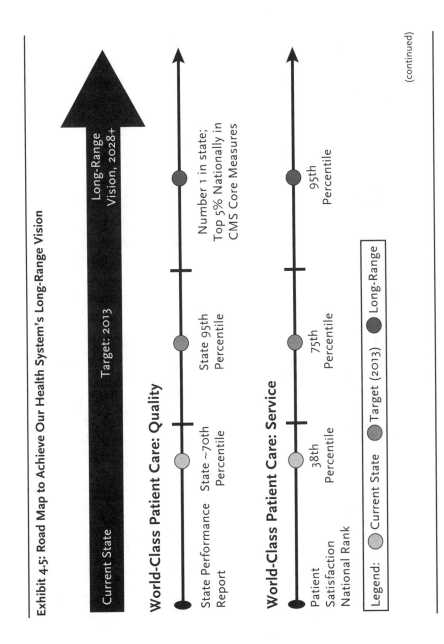

Current State

Target: 2013

Long-Range Vision, 2028+

World-Class Patient Care: Quality

State Performance Report

State ~70th Percentile

State 95th Percentile

Number 1 in state; Top 5% Nationally in CMS Core Measures

World-Class Patient Care: Service

Patient Satisfaction National Rank

38th Percentile

75th Percentile

95th Percentile

Legend: Current State Target (2013) Long-Range

(continued)

Exhibit 4-5: Road Map to Achieve Our Health System's Long-Range Vision

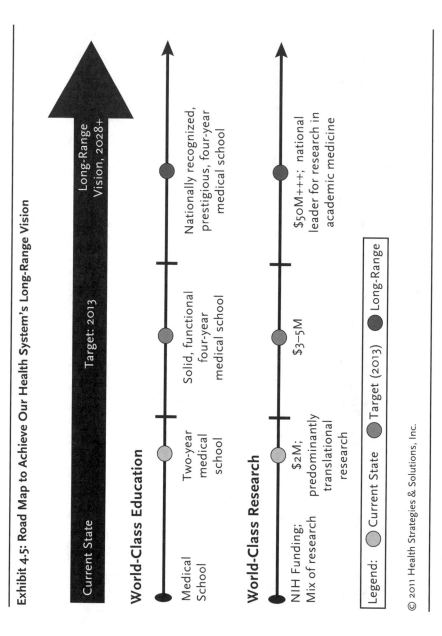

Current State

Target: 2013

Long-Range
Vision, 2028+

World-Class Education

Medical
School

Two-year
medical
school

Solid, functional
four-year
medical school

Nationally recognized,
prestigious, four-year
medical school

World-Class Research

NIH Funding;
Mix of research

$2M;
predominantly
translational
research

$3–5M

$50M+++; national
leader for research in
academic medicine

Legend: ⬤ Current State ⬤ Target (2013) ⬤ Long-Range

ning committee, and other key leaders should produce an effective vision statement without excessive attention to wordsmithery.

DEVELOPMENT OF OVERALL ORGANIZATION STRATEGY

The mission and vision address the why and what of future direction. Many healthcare organizations cannot or do not distinguish between the why/what and the how of future direction and inappropriately include strategy in mission or vision statements. They have difficulty determining a principal means (i.e., strategy) to accomplish the ends (i.e., mission and vision) they have articulated from those ends. Such an organization often sets forth multiple and diverse overall strategies, which compounds the confusion and results in no strategy at all.

Porter (1996) argues that many senior managers mistake operational effectiveness for strategy and as a result move away from viable competitive positions: "A major challenge for leadership is developing or reestablishing a clear strategy, not just improving operational effectiveness and making deals." The result: Overall organization strategy is often the least clearly defined element of future direction.

Strategy Development Frameworks

Miles and Snow (1978) developed a typology to describe a hospital's strategic orientation, classifying hospitals into four categories: prospectors, defenders, analyzers, and reactors.

- A *prospector* is defined as an organization that makes frequent changes in and additions to its services and markets and consistently responds rapidly to market opportunities by being the first to provide a new service or develop a new market.

- A *defender* offers a fairly stable set of services to defined markets and tends to ignore changes that do not directly affect current operations, focusing instead on doing its best in the current arena.
- An *analyzer*, like a defender, maintains a relatively stable base of services but selectively develops new services or markets like the prospector does. However, the analyzer rarely is the first to provide new services or expand into new markets, choosing instead to monitor actions of others and follow with a well thought out, thorough approach.
- A *reactor* is an organization that does not appear to respond consistently to changes in the market and seems to lack a coherent strategy. The reactor may, on occasion, be an early entrant into a new market or service but usually is forced into action by external events or after considerable evidence of potential for success.

A healthcare organization may have difficulty articulating its strategy as that of a defender, an analyzer, or a reactor. As Shortell, Morrison, and Friedman (1990) point out, many healthcare organizations espouse a prospector strategy, but few truly follow it, which may partly explain their confusion about overall strategy.

Another framework for overall strategy that is prevalent in general business, developed by Porter (1980), suggests that companies follow one of three principal strategies (singly or in combination) to create a defendable position: overall cost leadership, differentiation, or focus (also called niching).

The overall cost leadership strategy is achieved through a set of aggressive policies that ensure construction of efficient facilities, continuous pursuit of cost reduction, and systematic control of costs and overhead. Differentiation of a product or service offering means creating something that is perceived throughout the field as unique. The differentiation strategy does not ignore costs, but they are not the primary strategic focus. The focus strategy centers on a particular buyer or geographic market. While low-cost and differentiation strategies aim to establish the organization as a leader industrywide, the focus strategy aims to serve a particular target well, and policies are developed with this in mind. The organization is then able to serve its narrow target focus more effectively than those competing broadly.

Organization Strategy Characteristics

Hamel (1996) argues that successful strategy must be revolutionary: "Never has the world been more hospitable to industry revolutionaries and more hostile to industry incumbents." Hamel describes nine routes to industry revolution that involve reconceiving a product or service, redefining market space, and redrawing industry boundaries.

Regardless of which strategy framework it adopts, the organization must choose from among available alternative future strategies to have a high probability of realizing its vision. A principal strategy needs to be selected and articulated to all affected internal organizational constituencies as a key part of the organization's direction.

Exhibit 4.6 presents several examples of strategy statements from organizations inside and outside healthcare. Exhibit 4.7 shows the strategy statement developed in the BC Children's Hospital strategic plan referenced in Chapter 3 and relates it to the companion mission and vision statements. Examples of clear healthcare strategy statements are difficult to find because so few organizations, especially not-for-profits, pursue any discernible strategy. Many are still on the rebound from the trendy strategy of the 1990s—integration—and of the first decade of the twenty-first century—refocusing on the core business. Opportunism and drift, rather than strategy, seem to be the norm today.

Exhibit 4.6: Strategy Statement Examples

Non-healthcare
Procter & Gamble: Product excellence
Nordstrom: Service to the customer

Healthcare
Ascension Health, St. Louis, Missouri, "Strategic Direction": We will fulfill our promise to those we serve by delivering Healthcare That Works, Healthcare That Is Safe, and Healthcare That Leaves No One Behind, for life
Community Health Systems, Brentwood, Tennessee, "The CHS Business Model": Effectively integrating organizations and improving hospital operations

Exhibit 4.7: BC Children's Hospital Organizational Direction Statement

Our Mission	Our Vision	Our Overall Strategy
Why do we exist?	What we are striving to do?	How we will get there?
We care, educate, discover, and advocate to improve the health of children and youth	To transform child and youth health	Serve as a catalyst for change in the child and youth health system

Source: BC Children's Hospital, 2009. Used with permission.

Organization Strategy Development Process

The process of developing overall organization strategy is similar to that described earlier for the mission and vision statements. The main difference is in the degree to which the strategy statement emanates from planning staff and top management versus the strategic planning committee and the board.

DEVELOPMENT OF THE VALUES STATEMENT

The values statement is the underpinning of the entire organizational direction and strategic plan. Like the mission statement, the values statement is widely disseminated to internal and external constituencies. In the absence of significant organizational or environmental changes, this statement is relatively timeless and may not require major modification.

With the proliferation of mergers and other forms of affiliation; the growth of integrated delivery systems; and, for some, disaffiliation and disintegration, few healthcare organizations have been untouched by the waves of change sweeping the industry. In these new, larger organizations, diverse cultures are brought together, and existing values are blended into, or in some cases imposed on, the new entity. The core of the values statement is a representation of the desired character of the new organizational culture and sets forth the manner in which that character is conveyed to employees and other stakeholders. As some organizations downsize, restructure, and divest themselves of component parts, the values of the surviving entities often must be reexamined.

In stable, successful healthcare organizations a values statement can be gleaned from organizational behavior. Observance of the day-to-day practices of the employees and of board policy and performance will lead to a fairly clear picture of the organization's values. This values statement can be fine-tuned by leadership to reflect some minor modification of organization behavior and then serve as the product of the values definition task.

For other healthcare organizations, such as brand new organizations, those with high organic growth, or those in rapid organic decline, a values statement should be developed through a top-down process similar to that recommended for the mission state-

Exhibit 4.8: Values Statement Examples

Non-healthcare
Disney Corporation
• No cynicism
• Nurturing and promulgation of "wholesome American values"
• Creativity, dreams, and imagination
• Fanatical attention to consistency and detail
• Preservation and control of the Disney image

Healthcare
Memorial Health System, Springfield, Illinois
• Service to Humanity
• Excellence in Performance
• Respect for the Individual
• Value of Employees
• Integrity in Relationships
• Community Responsibility
• Equal Access

ment. Where current organizational values are determined to be inadequate or not conducive to providing high-quality healthcare and new or significantly different organizational values must be instituted, leadership must discover how the existing values came into being. Then the organization must conduct a self-examination to create a new values statement for the future.

An example of a recently developed values statement, typical of what many healthcare organizations aspire to, is illustrated in Exhibit 4.8. Note, as well, the Disney Corporation values statement, and given the general public knowledge of this organization, how tailored and descriptive a values statement can be.

CONCLUSION

Four critical outputs—mission, vision, strategy, and values state-ments—constitute the product of organizational direction and are developed during activity II of the strategic planning process. With direction identified, productive movement into the next level of detail in strategic planning—strategy formulation, made up of major initiatives, goals, and objectives, to address the important issues outlined in activity I—may now begin.

As the organization moves further into the how of strategic planning, the roles and responsibilities of management expand. The board, both directly and through its strategic planning com-mittee, may have had significant input into the organizational direction because it represents the major policy elements of the strategic plan; with the completion of the organizational direction activities, the transition from board-driven strategic planning to staff-driven strategic planning begins.

CHAPTER 5

Activity III: Strategy Formulation

The only constant in our business is that everything is changing. We have to take advantage of change and not let it take advantage of us. We have to be ahead of the game.

—*Michael Dell*

Strategy renders choices about what not to do as important as choices about what to do.

—*Michael Porter*

FROM VISION TO GOALS

Once leaders have defined the overall direction of their organization, they can turn to determining its goals, objectives, and future strategic development. As emphasized in Chapter 4, significant progress must be made in a number of key areas to achieve the vision of the next five to ten years. Exhibit 5.1 shows the critical relationship between organizational direction and strategy formulation and defines the outputs of each strategic planning activity.

Exhibit 5.2 highlights a few especially important points about the strategy formulation phase of strategic planning. Broadening the number and type of internal participants involved in plan development and bringing multiple diverse perspectives to bear on strategy formulation are desirable tasks to undertake. In large,

Exhibit 5.1: From Organizational Direction to Strategy Formulation

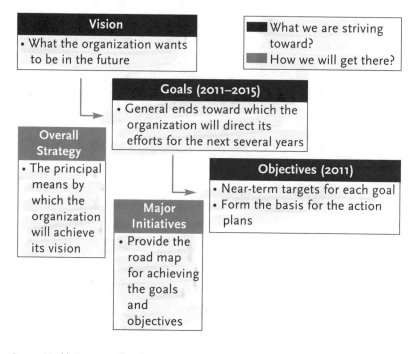

© 2011 Health Strategies & Solutions, Inc.

multi-entity organizations, strategy formulation usually begins at the system or corporate level and the framework developed is then used for operating unit or other strategy formulation.

For many organizations, the most difficult part of strategic planning is moving from the vision to the next level of detail: the goals. Identifying hundreds of goals that support the vision is tempting but should be avoided, as it results in an unwieldy plan that cannot be implemented. Healthcare organizations also struggle with setting measurable, clear goals, tending instead to specify a series of activities or processes or a vague directional intent (e.g., "improve quality"). This chapter addresses these problems directly.

Strategic planning at its essence is the process of making difficult choices from among competing priorities and focusing the orga-

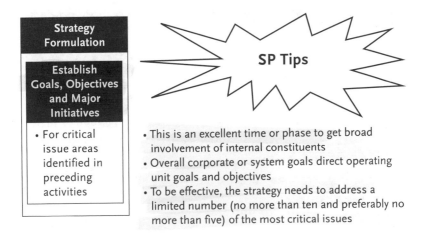

Strategy Formulation

Establish Goals, Objectives and Major Initiatives

SP Tips

- For critical issue areas identified in preceding activities

- This is an excellent time or phase to get broad involvement of internal constituents
- Overall corporate or system goals direct operating unit goals and objectives
- To be effective, the strategy needs to address a limited number (no more than ten and preferably no more than five) of the most critical issues

© 2011 Health Strategies & Solutions, Inc.

nization's limited resources on the areas that will yield the greatest payoff. For strategic planning to be effective, that focus must be maintained throughout the process—and especially in this transition from vision to goals. Successful organizations identify only a small set of goals that are imperatives for realizing the vision—preferably no more than five, and certainly no more than ten.

Moving from vision to goals is most readily accomplished through a three-phase process:

1. Determine critical issues
2. Prepare white papers on critical issues
3. Identify goals

Determining Critical Issues

Critical issues are determined by examining the organization's mission, vision, and key organizational strategy in light of the initial

Exhibit 5.3: The Strategy Formulation Process

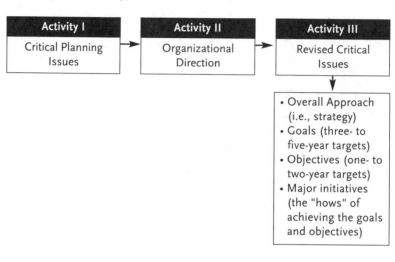

issues defined in the environmental assessment (see Exhibit 5.3). Often the issues the organization defined in activity I survive largely intact as its final set of critical issues. Sometimes the issues may need to be reshaped because of conclusions reached in the organizational direction phase.

Determining what constitutes a critical issue is clearly subjective, and healthcare executives are commonly confused by this step. Typically, critical issues stand out as central to achieving the vision, have a deep potential impact on the organization, and cannot be addressed easily or resolved in the short term. Another commonly made distinction is that these issues deal primarily with concerns outside the realm of day-to-day operations.

One of two approaches is typically used to determine the final list of critical issues. The more process-intensive approach, used most often when the initial list of issues is large or controversial, consists of three steps. First, each member of the strategic planning committee identifies the top three or so issues and a master list is compiled. Assuming the priorities are not obvious from this first

Exhibit 5.4: Critical Issues

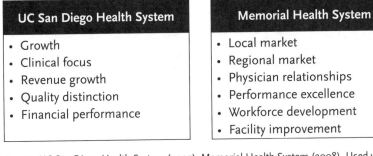

UC San Diego Health System	Memorial Health System
• Growth	• Local market
• Clinical focus	• Regional market
• Revenue growth	• Physician relationships
• Quality distinction	• Performance excellence
• Financial performance	• Workforce development
	• Facility improvement

Source: UC San Diego Health System (2007); Memorial Health System (2008). Used with permission.

step, a second step is to have some discussion of what each issue is and why it is important. Some issues may fall off the list or be consolidated as a result. Third, the committee members are asked to vote for the top three issues; the most frequently named issues make the final list.

The second approach is for planning staff or a small group of senior management to narrow the number of potential issues down to no more than ten and present the findings of their analyses to the strategic planning committee for review and modification. It is important to specify why the selected areas are strategically significant and why other areas are not. Two representative lists of critical issues that resulted from such a process are shown in Exhibit 5.4.

Preparing White Papers on Critical Issues

Once critical issues are identified, the focus moves from issues to goals. A process-intensive approach is most likely to identify the best goals, objectives, major initiatives, and actions and build support for plan implementation and action. The more process-intensive the approach, the more time required to complete it.

A highly intensive approach can take as long as two or three months, while the least intensive approach can be completed in as little as three or four weeks. If the time frame for planning is a concern, the approach selected for this activity should be carefully considered.

Leaders can choose from three basic paths to transition to goal setting:

1. **Move directly from critical issues to goals**. Planning staff, senior management, or the strategic planning committee develop the goals without further analysis or process.
2. **Prepare white papers on critical issues**. Preparing these in-depth reports helps distinguish and prioritize alternatives. Planning staff prepare position papers on each issue and recommend goals for review and modification by senior management and the strategic planning committee.
3. **Convene task forces to prepare white papers**. This option is similar to option 2, except that a multidisciplinary group of organizational representatives convenes for a limited period to assist in preparing the white papers.

The task force alternative has an additional benefit: It exposes important organizational stakeholders to the outline of the burgeoning strategic plan and constructively engages them in further definition of organizational strategy in areas that are personally significant and relevant. A few guidelines, presented in the following paragraphs, can help organizations to manage this third path.

Assemble the Task Forces with Care
No foolproof formula exists for assembling task forces, but recognizing all the ends the organization is trying to accomplish and the potential incompatibility of those ends is a good starting point. A typical set of principles for task force composition includes these:

- Gain broad representation from potentially affected constituencies *[handwritten: i.e. talk about doctors need does on taskforce]*
- Include enough diversity so that the task force is not biased toward any single perspective
- Achieve relatively good chemistry among the members
- Keep the group small enough that it is not unwieldy
- Select members who are interested enough to participate actively
- Choose a leader who will lead, but not dominate

The task forces typically will meet three to four times over a six- to eight-week (or longer) period. The members should understand and appreciate that their charge is time limited and that they are not making decisions, only presenting alternatives and making recommendations to the strategic planning committee.

Give Task Forces Guidelines and Support

Although active participation and free-flowing discussion are to be encouraged, some structure and staff support are necessary to achieve sound outputs and leave the participants feeling that they were constructively involved in the process. Expectations of the task forces need to be defined clearly at the outset, including time frame for deliberation, questions to answer or issues to address, and likely structure of the output needed. Exhibits 5.5 and 5.6 give samples of guidance that might be provided to task forces. Appendix 5.1 presents an example of a full white paper developed using this outline. Data and other relevant information collected in earlier planning activities should be assembled and provided to task force members before their first meeting. The planning staff should be introduced as staff support to the task forces and play a major role in logistical support, data support, and production of the white papers.

Exhibit 5.5: Task Force Overview

Strategic Issue	Issues to be Explored	Proposed Leadership and Membership Profile

1. Primary care network	• Size and distribution of the network
	• Operational and financial expectations
	• Mechanisms for incorporating physicians into the network
		• Leader: Primary care physician
		• Members:
		  – Managed care marketing staff
		  – Senior management
		  – Practice managers

2. Cost position	• Cost target required to compete successfully
	• Schedule to attain targeted costs
	• Approaches to cost management and reduction
		• Leader: Chief financial officer
		• Members:
		  – Department chairs
		  – Senior management

3. Medical education	• Role of medical education within system
	• Expectations of medical education and criteria for evaluating residencies
	• Need for an academic affiliation
		• Leader: Teaching physician
		• Members:
		  – Physicians trained at system programs
		  – Other physicians
		  – Senior management

Source: Pinnacle Health System (1996). Used with permission.

Exhibit 5.6: White Paper Outline

- Issue definition
- Background (including importance of resolving the issue)
- Qualitative and quantitative description of situation
- Strategies being employed by others faced with similar situations
- Options available, pros and cons, evaluation of options
- Recommended option(s) to pursue
- Major goals for a three- to five-year planning horizon; objectives for next year (or two); major initiatives (categories of activities) to achieve goals and objectives
- Barriers and constraints to achieving goals and objectives

© 2011 Health Strategies & Solutions, Inc.

Exhibit 5.7: Wayne Memorial Health System Critical Issues: Current and Desired State

	Poor	Fair	Good	Excellent
Physician retention/ recruitment		O———————————————————→●		
Emergency services	O—————————————————————————————→●			
Quality and service			O———————————————→●	
Breadth and depth of services			O———————————————→●	
Fiscal responsibility				O————→●

LEGEND: O Current state ● Desired state

Source: Wayne Memorial Health System (2008). Used with permission.

Identifying Goals

Ideally, each white paper will thoroughly review all aspects of the critical issues it addresses and present recommendations that allow a goal, or, occasionally, multiple goals, to be readily identified. It is the strategic planning committee's job to select a goal that will con-

Exhibit 5.8: Wayne Memorial Health System (WMHS) Critical Issues and Goals

Critical Issues	FY2008–FY2013 Goals
Physician retention/ recruitment	WMHS has 50% larger and more stable (< 5% annual turnover) base of quality primary care physicians and specialists actively practicing at WMHS.
Emergency department	WMHS ED satisfaction ranks in the 90th percentile in patient satisfaction and performs much better than industry norms for efficiency and turnaround.
Quality and service	WMHS performs better than regional competitors on publicly available quality comparisons and outperforms them on patient satisfaction.
Breadth and depth of services	At least 40% to 45% of service area residents choose WMHS for care (versus 31% inpatient market share in 2006).
Fiscal responsibility	WMHS sustains an operating margin (≥ 3%) and access to capital (as measured by cash on hand and debt/capitalization ratio) sufficient to continue investment in the growth and development of the organization in a financially prudent manner.

Source: Wayne Memorial Health System (2008). Used with permission.

structively and creatively deal with the critical issue and be potentially useful in achieving part of the vision.

Typically, each task force leader presents the team's report to the strategic planning committee for review, modification, and, ultimately, acceptance. A goal is then identified, discussed, and modified before the strategic planning committee approves it. Exhibits 5.7 and 5.8 show the relationship between critical issues and goals.

Note that the goals have been stated in measurable forms, whenever possible, and as targets to be achieved in the future— they are essentially "what" statements rather than "how." Goals

Exhibit 5.9: Our Health System (OHS) Strategy Recommendations

Goals, 2013	Major Initiatives, 2008–2013
• OHS scores in the top 5% of [state] hospitals for quality performance • OHS's signature programs have superior recognition in southern [state] and compete with metro area-based AMCs	• Achieve highest rankings or ratings on public quality measures • Define and develop three to five signature programs (centers of excellence) • Invest in cutting-edge technology, as feasible, to differentiate signature programs • Recruit superstar physicians to differentiate signature programs • Leverage academic excellence in signature programs
Objectives, 2008–2009	
• Quality outcome scores are in the top 15% of [state] hospitals • Two signature programs are recognized as superior to any other southern [state] provider	

© 2011 Health Strategies & Solutions, Inc.

Exhibit 5.10: Example Prioritization of Five-Year Initiatives

High	• Expand primary care network • Continue performance excellence journey • Execute long-range facility plan • Expand workforce development
Medium	• Strengthen clinic relationships • Grow university relationships • Develop centers of excellence • Build ambulatory care clinics • Consider modifying scope of services • Enhance appeal to physicians
Low	• Collaborate with hospital-based physicians • Establish stronger presence in county • Expedite transfers and referrals

Note: High-priority initiatives receive 75% of resources in implementation; medium-priority initiatives receive 20% of resources in implementation (some may need to be deferred); low-priority initiatives receive 5% of resources in implementation (very modest effort or deferral required).

© 2011 Health Strategies & Solutions, Inc.

and objectives should be framed as ends to be achieved on the way to the vision, leaving how to achieve them to be determined by the major initiatives and the tactical details in the action plan. An example of the relationship among the three major outputs of strategy formulation—goals, objectives, and major initiatives—from a medical center strategic plan is shown in Exhibit 5.9.

Typically, the result of the task force/strategy formulation process is the identification of 10 to 20 major initiatives for the organization to pursue in implementing its strategic plan. Because organizations rarely have the resources to pursue so many initiatives vigorously and equally, the strategic planning committee may need to prioritize the initiatives. An example of prioritization during a regional referral center's creation of a strategic plan is shown in Exhibit 5.10. Such a prioritization process will help set the stage for a realistic and achievable implementation plan. The completion of goals and major initiative setting is significant in that it puts in place the final piece of the strategic plan with which the board should be principally concerned. Collectively, the mission, vision, strategy, values, goals, and major initiatives constitute the strategic portion of the plan, whereas the remaining components—objectives and actions—are more tactical and operational. It may be helpful to think about the strategic plan as composed of two parts: strategy, which has been the subject of chapters 4 and 5 until this point, and the management action plan, which remains to be completed.

Few not-for-profit boards understand or appreciate the distinction between the strategic and tactical parts of the process. Although the work of the strategic planning committee as a whole should be wrapped up at this point and management should take responsibility for completing the remaining plan tasks and components, most strategic planning committees continue to function in an increasingly dysfunctional way until the plan is complete.

In this situation, a compromise may be in order. Rather than finish the committee's work at this point or allow the committee to continue to provide similar oversight as in prior tasks, the senior management team should thank the committee for completing the overwhelming majority of its important work and offer to reconvene it when the objectives and actions are drafted. Management can then present its draft management action plan and an executive summary of the plan to the committee. Following the committee's review, the action plan and executive summary are submitted to the full board for approval and adoption.

ESTABLISHING OBJECTIVES

If the suggested approach is followed, the remaining planning tasks are carried out under the direction of senior management. These tasks typically involve broader representation of management team members than has been the case up to this point.

Essentially, each goal needs to be dissected into smaller, more manageable components:

- **Objectives**—short-term targets in each goal area
- **Actions**—the principal activities that need to be accomplished to achieve the objectives (and relate to parts of the major initiatives)

The objectives and actions (the latter discussed in Chapter 6) collectively compose the near-term game plan to move the organization's strategic plan forward.

Sometimes the objectives are well developed in the white papers and task force discussions. In other cases, senior management staff need to determine the objectives, individually or collectively. In either event, the objectives need to provide intermediate, preferably measurable targets on the path to achieving the goals. Review the example of goals and related objectives of one organization shown earlier in Exhibit 5.9.

CONTINGENCY PLANNING

It is helpful to step back once or twice during the strategic planning process to consider how the expected direction and strategy will hold up under the likely alternative future conditions identified at the end of the environmental assessment. Some contingent events may be incorporated explicitly in the strategy formulation process for specific goals and objectives resulting from the barriers and constraints analysis mentioned in Exhibit 5.6. Other more macro environmental possibilities could affect a broad range of strategy formulation outcomes.

Typical contingencies to consider today include the following:

- Implementation of healthcare reform initiatives
- Major economic change, such as a deep and prolonged recession
- Restructuring of the local or regional environment, such as consolidation and merger and acquisition activity
- Effects of natural disasters

An example of contingency planning and its impact on the full range of preliminarily defined goals and objectives is illustrated in Exhibit 5.11. In this case, six significant contingencies were examined: one major federal policy change, one major state policy change, and four changes involving local or regional market dynamics. As a result, the senior management team and the board felt that all reasonable scenarios had been considered and plan implementation moved forward expeditiously and with their full confidence, but with greater ability to adapt should conditions change during implementation.

FINANCIAL ANALYSIS

One final topic in strategy formulation deserves discussion. Great controversy exists among strategic planners and other healthcare executives about the appropriate depth and breadth of financial

Exhibit 5.11: Contingency Planning: National Health Reform (from mid-2008 Strategic Plan)

Description	Likelihood	Warning Signs	Implications for System	Readiness/Actions
• Model depends on both political and economic factors • Anticipate phased approach, beginning with extension of coverage to the uninsured with low to medium incomes • May include multistate demonstration projects • Increased regulation to discourage unnecessary use and incentives to address obvious problems such as chronic care • Emphasis on consumer-directed healthcare (HSAs)	• Low to moderate in next five years	• A Democratic president and Democratic majorities in both houses of Congress • Continued pressure to make health insurance affordable even in a resurgent economy • Severe economic distress that increases the number of uninsured • Significant cuts in provider revenue that cause some hospitals to fail and increase pressure for a government bailout • Continuation of dramatic decline in employer-sponsored coverage	• Will force movement from high-margin areas to underserved areas • Greater financial risk to small system hospitals with the exception of some safety net services • Patient safety and outcome criteria will affect both volume and reimbursement	• Improve readiness by building up outpatient business, though this will not optimize revenue in the near term • Ensure systems are in place for managing care, reducing costs of poor quality, reducing variation, and identifying and implementing best practices • Develop a more comprehensive system that improves efficiency and reduces costs • Evaluate current and future impact of HSAs on service lines

Source: Memorial Health System (2008). Used with permission.

analysis in the strategic planning process. A minimalist approach is recommended in this book; however, other texts promote the belief that something close to a financial feasibility forecast is necessary.

Current thinking on financial analysis in strategic planning, as embodied in much of the literature referenced in Chapter 1, is consistent with the approach recommended here. For example, Bellenfant and Nelson (2002) suggest that the financial analysis in strategic planning should be "a reality check, ensuring that an organization's strategies do not outstrip its resources and that new initiatives provide the desired level of value." Nonetheless, because a wide range of perspectives exist, a few examples are provided in Appendixes 5.2 and 5.3.

The strategic plan should have a high-level strategy focus; any substantial financial analysis should occur in implementation or later. However, one note of caution is important. The approach recommended in this book is one that is continually vigilant in recognizing resource limitations, making choices, and focusing effort. This approach can be accomplished with a process that has financial awareness and concerns as parts of its infrastructure so that financial implications are implicitly part of each step of the process. If such high awareness and astuteness is not routinely part of the organization's work, some substantive financial tasks may need to be included in the strategic planning process.

CONCLUSION

When activity III is complete, the organization will have a sound framework, through its goals, major initiatives, and objectives, for the work that lies ahead in implementing the plan. But, even more important, if the planning process has been successfully carried out, one of its by-products will be shared learning among organizational leaders about how to address each critical issue. Consensus or near consensus on managing these issues will facilitate problem-free approval of the strategic plan and a rapid transition from planning to implementation.

Example White Paper

ISSUE DEFINITION AND BACKGROUND AND SITUATION DESCRIPTION

> Community Medical Center (CMC) has made some effort to develop clinical areas of expertise but has not developed a true center of excellence (COE). Without some level of COE development, CMC services will not be differentiated in the market.

- CMC offers a broad scope of clinical services. Current programmatic strengths include cardiovascular, orthopedics, women's health, and behavioral health.
- Regional Hospital is an aggressive system offering similar clinical services that directly compete with CMC's.

- Collaborative and successful working relationships with University Hospital could strengthen service lines and contribute to development of COEs.
- Projected population growth over the next five years is minimal, and market growth will be modest; therefore, competition will be among hospitals in service lines.

STRATEGIES EMPLOYED BY OTHERS

Hospitals like CMC that have been successful in developing COEs have concentrated on developing a limited number of them—one to three total at any point in time. Hospitals that have attempted to develop multiple COEs have not succeeded because of the extremely high degree of resources required in each area of COE development.

- Nationally, major medical centers are moving toward developing COEs.
- Many COEs being developed are comprehensive and offer a multidisciplinary approach to care.
- While many systems attempt to develop multiple COEs, *successful* systems develop a limited number (one to three) initially.
- Given minimal population growth in CMC's primary service area, outreach to the secondary service area will be important in COE development.
- Linkage to clinical research and clinical trial opportunities appeals to today's informed consumer.
- Community hospital COEs benefit from relationships with academic health systems like University Hospital.

OPTIONS AVAILABLE TO CMC

The planning committee considered the options available to CMC. Based on market conditions and the need to develop some areas of distinction for CMC, it was decided that CMC should strive to create one to three highly developed COEs while offering quality services across the remaining clinical areas.

Options	Pros and Cons of Options
• Do not develop a true COE; strive to be good across all CMC clinical services. • Create one to three highly developed COEs and offer quality services across the remaining clinical areas. • Focus on developing many COEs.	• Increasingly, providers must offer points of distinction from competitors. • COE development has a halo effect on other hospital services. • Developing multiple COEs is extremely resource intensive.

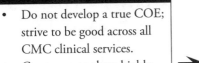

CMC'S PROPOSED STRATEGY

The proposed strategy calls for CMC to develop COEs; however, the number of COEs will be limited to only a few over the next five years. Given current quality and performance, cardio-vascular services could be quickly and efficiently positioned in the marketplace as a comprehensive, multidisciplinary COE for CMC. It is also proposed that additional COEs be developed over time and new services be created to meet market need.

Recommendation

- Aggressively continue the development of cardiovascular services as a COE.
- Continue to roll out the development of other COEs such as orthopedics, women's health, and behavioral health.
- Identify and strengthen other key clinical services by determining those with the greatest likelihood of success in the market, including ability to meet market demand, potential to be a market leader and develop selective niches for CMC, and rational use of resources.
- Develop the strongest possible synergistic clinical relationships with University Hospital.

Goals (2009 to 2014)

- CMC is the leading regional provider of cardiovascular services and is recognized for its COEs in one to two additional clinical programs.

Objectives (2009 to 2014)

- Cardiovascular services is a comprehensive, multidisciplinary COE.
- Key elements required to become a successful COE are in place for one to two additional programs (potentially orthopedics, women's health, behavioral health, pediatrics, or oncology).
- Routine programmatic improvements continue in emergency department and trauma, neurosciences, and other services.
- Other clinical services are identified and significantly enhanced on the basis of market need and opportunity; services considered for enhancement include digestive diseases, geriatrics, and health and wellness.

Measurement Criteria

- Quality indicators
- Volume and market position
- Financial performance
- Differentiation from competitors (consumer image)

CMC'S BARRIERS AND CONSTRAINTS

- Extremely formidable competition from Regional Hospital in cardiovascular services
- Capital needs given financial position and competing priorities
- Lacking leadership to drive COE development outside of cardiovascular services

EXAMPLE: STRATEGIC FINANCIAL ANALYSIS
PROJECTED BASELINE INCOME STATEMENT

	Budgeted FY2009	Projected FY2014
Revenue	$492,230	$599,460
Expenses	$495,840	$601,260
Operating income	$ (3,610)	$(1,800)
Operating margin	−0.73%	−0.30%
Non-operating gains	$4,930	$6,290
Net income	$1,320	$4,490
Net margin	0.27%	0.75%

Note: Dollars in 000's.

EXAMPLE: NET FINANCIAL IMPACT FROM MAJOR INITIATIVES

	FY2009	FY2010	FY2011	FY2012	FY2013	FY2014	Net Impact from Major Initiatives
Baseline net income	$1.3M	$1.5M	$2.1M	$2.8M	$3.6M	$4.5M	
Estimated Impact from Major Initiatives							
IP volume growth	$0.3M	$0.6M	$0.9M	$1.2M	$1.4M	$1.6M	$6.0M
Ambulatory surgery volume growth	$0.0M	$0.1M	$0.1M	$0.1M	$0.2M	$0.2M	$0.7M
Program/service closures	$0.5M	$0.9M	$1.4M	$1.8M	$2.0M	$2.4M	$9.0M
Increased commitment of community physicians	$0.5M	$0.9M	$1.4M	$1.8M	$2.0M	$2.4M	$9.0M
Expense reduction	$0.5M	$1.5M	$2.2M	$2.2M	$2.2M	$2.2M	$10.8M
Quality investment	($0.8M)	($0.8M)	($0.8M)	($0.8M)	($0.8M)	($0.8M)	($4.8M)
Revised net income	$2.3M	$4.7M	$7.3M	$9.1M	$10.6M	$12.5M	

© 2011 Health Strategies & Solutions, Inc.

EXAMPLE: STRATEGIC FINANCIAL ANALYSIS
PROGRAM/SERVICE REDUCTION CRITERIA

CHS should use specific criteria when considering which programs or services to discontinue, downsize, or restructure.

Criteria	Positive (+)	Neutral (o)	Negative (−)
Market size	Large	Medium	Small
CHS market position	Strong	Moderate	Weak
CHS clinical competency	Strong	Moderate	Weak
Competition	Limited	Moderate	Strong
Payer mix	Excellent	Good	Poor
Profitability	High	Moderate	Low
Alignment with core business	High	Moderate	Low

EXAMPLE: PRELIMINARY ANALYSIS OF EXISTING PROGRAMS/ SERVICES TO DISCONTINUE, REDUCE, OR RESTRUCTURE

	IP Pediatrics	IP Psych	Health Center	ASC
Market size	Medium (~3K discharge)	Large (>5K cases)	Medium	Large (>40K cases)
CHS market position	Weak (share = 7%)	Weak (share = 19%)	Strong (Occ >90%)	Weak (share <15%)
CHS clinical competency	Weak	Strong	Strong	Moderate
Competition	Strong	Moderate	Moderate	Strong
Payer mix	Poor	Poor	Poor	Good
Profitability (×2)[a]	Low (loss –$0.2M)	Low (loss –$7.8M)	Low (loss –$1.4M)	Low (loss –$0.5M)
Alignment with core business	Moderate	Moderate	Moderate	High
Preliminary recommendation	Discontinue	Discontinue or restructure	Discontinue or restructure	Discontinue or restructure

(a) Weight is twice that of other criteria.

Note: ASC = ambulatory surgery center

© 2011 Health Strategies & Solutions, Inc.

CHAPTER 6

Activity IV: Transitioning to Implementation

When it comes to getting things done, we need fewer
architects and more bricklayers.

—*Colleen C. Barrett*

Never mistake motion for action.

—*Ernest Hemingway*

While developing a good strategic plan is not easy, implementation is far more difficult. And, the transition from strategic planning to implementation is a point where plans have the potential to set the stage for implementation success, or more typically, where efforts stray off course.

A study conducted by this author of the state of the art in healthcare strategic planning in 2005-2006 (Zuckerman 2007) revealed that while the core strategic plan development tasks were perceived by senior leaders as being carried out well or very well, implementation planning, implementation itself, and communication of the strategic plan inside and outside of the organization were cited as areas in which significant improvement can and should occur.

Exhibit 6.1 identifies some of the key elements of this final activity of the strategic planning process and highlights: (1) the

Exhibit 6.1: Developing the Plan: Action Planning

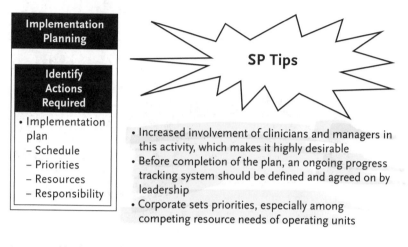

Implementation Planning	SP Tips
Identify Actions Required	

• Implementation plan
  – Schedule
  – Priorities
  – Resources
  – Responsibility
	• Increased involvement of clinicians and managers in this activity, which makes it highly desirable
	• Before completion of the plan, an ongoing progress tracking system should be defined and agreed on by leadership
	• Corporate sets priorities, especially among competing resource needs of operating units

importance of increased involvement of those who will be principal participants in implementation of the plan; (2) the need to specify and adhere to an ongoing tracking system for plan implementation; and (3) the critical role in larger healthcare systems of the corporate organization in defining and mediating demands for resources required to carry out implementation.

Here are a few comments on the key subcomponents:

- **Assignment of responsibilities for implementation**. Specific individuals must be designated and held accountable for each objective and action.
- **Communications and roll out**. A formal, highly inclusive, and informative roll out of the strategic plan should assist in facilitating implementation.
- **Detailed planning**. In certain cases, more detailed analysis or study during the implementation phase may be desirable and warranted and should be anticipated, structured, and managed.

- **Monitoring progress**. Progress must be monitored on a regular basis during implementation, with plans adjusted as needed.
- **Regular plan review and update**. If at all possible, the organization should commit to carrying out strategic planning on an ongoing basis.

IMPLEMENTATION FRAMEWORK

The last substantive strategic planning task is the preparation of an implementation framework. This task involves taking the objectives identified as the final output in Chapter 5 and putting them into a framework that facilitates implementation and ongoing monitoring of implementation progress. At a minimum, actions for each objective need to be developed, and each action should be assigned to a primary party who will be responsible for directing and scheduling implementation.

Some implementation frameworks include additional information such as secondary parties or groups who will support implementation, incremental operational or capital resource requirements and time frame approval requirements, significant decision-making needs, and timing. A basic implementation framework is illustrated in Exhibit 6.2, and an example implementation plan appears in Exhibit 6.3.

When implementation nears, the typical strategic planning process involves additional members of the healthcare organization's management team. As noted earlier, during the course of the strategic plan development process, primary responsibility shifts from the board, whose focus is on the early strategic policy recommendations, to the senior management, whose responsibility it will be to implement these policies and provide consistent strategic direction to all the operational entities of the organization, and finally to a broad group of middle management and staff who will act as the frontline implementation team.

Exhibit 6.2: Sample Implementation Format

	Resource Requirements	Target Completion	Responsibility
Goal 1:	Magnitude of resources required ($ and effort)	Month and year (can also provide start date and key intermediate points)	Individual leading effort and support staff or team
1.1 Objective: a. b. c. d. e.			
1.2 Objective: a. b. c. d. e.			
1.3 Objective: a. b. c. d. e.			

The implementation team members need to understand the aspects of the strategic plan that have been developed largely by the board and senior management, and they need to actively participate in shaping those parts of the plan for which they will be principally responsible (i.e., actions, budget, and schedule). At this point in the process, broad-based involvement of middle managers and others is not only appropriate but critical.

Exhibit 6.3: Community Medical Center Action Plan: Clinical Excellence Through Service Line Development

GOAL: CMC is the leading regional provider of cardiovascular services and is recognized for its centers of excellence (COEs) in one to two additional clinical programs	Measurement Criteria: • Quality indicators • Volume and market position • Financial performance • Differentiation from competitors		
Objectives and Action Steps	Resource Requirements	Target Completion	Responsibility
1.1 Cardiovascular services is a comprehensive, multidisciplinary COE			Dr. S.
a. Analyze current programs and services to identify any gaps in services and ensure that CMC's cardiovascular program is comprehensive and multidisciplinary in nature	< $25,000	December 2009	
• Consider developing new programs such as extended care, congestive heart failure, and lipid clinic			
• Identify resource needs and requirements as well as return on investment (ROI)			
b. Review and revise current proposed facility plan that develops cardiovascular services as "hospital in a hospital" and moves all inpatient services into a contiguous area	$3.0 million	December 2009	
• Prioritize space relocation (consider developing reception area first, remodeling 3A, etc.)			
• In conjunction with facility plan, conduct a bed-need study to determine utilization and streamline efficiencies (e.g., observation beds in emergency department for patients from chest pain center)			
c. Conduct (an equipment) needs assessment and upgrade equipment	$2.5 million to $4.5 million	December 2010	
• Consider cath lab replacement, electrophysiology upgrades, additional monitored beds, fixed cath labs in emergency department			
d. Assess feasibility of implementing a nursing and allied health staffing plan based on projected volume growth, potential for dedicated staff (e.g., physical therapy, nutrition), and cross-training	< $25,000	December 2010	
e. Measure and monitor quality indicators and report on a regular basis	< $25,000	June 2010	

(continued)

Exhibit 6.3: Community Medical Center Action Plan: Clinical Excellence Through Service Line Development

GOAL: CMC is the leading regional provider of cardiovascular services and is recognized for its centers of excellence (COEs) in one to two additional clinical programs	**Measurement Criteria:** • Quality indicators • Volume and market position • Financial performance • Differentiation from competitors		
Objectives and Action Steps	Resource Requirements	Target Completion	Responsibility
f. Develop a comprehensive marketing plan (see infrastructure goal)	Refer to infrastructure	June 2010	
g. Develop a plan that enhances programmatic relationships with University Hospital	< $25,000	Ongoing	
h. Work with medical staff office to continue building physician relationships locally and regionally	< $25,000	Ongoing	
i. Establish a financial performance system that monitors financial indicators and measures ROI	< $25,000	June 2010	
1.2 Key elements required to become a successful COE are in place for one to two additional programs (potentially orthopedics, women's health, behavioral health, pediatrics, or oncology)			N. Jones
a. Establish a decision-making process to assist in identifying one to two additonal COEs			
• Define key elements required to be a COE (consider adding to those in CMC strategic plan)		December 2009	
• Build a financial model to assess proposed financial performance and ROI			
• Consider "redefining" COEs (e.g., orthopedics broadened to restorative care)			
b. Reassess orthopedics as a COE	TBD	June 2010	
c. Assess all other potential COEs (women's health, behavioral health, pediatrics, cancer, new program development) using the established decision-making process to identify an additional comprehensive COE	< $25,000	December 2010	

(continued)

Exhibit 6.3: Community Medical Center Action Plan: Clinical Excellence Through Service Line Development

	Resource Requirements	Target Completion	Responsibility
1.3 Routine programmatic improvements continue in emergency department and trauma, neurosciences, and other services	$50,000	December 2009	J. Williams
a. Complete emergency department and trauma certification process	TBD	Ongoing	
b. Continue neurosciences program development			
• Consider adding intensive care unit beds for neuro/trauma (incorporate into facilities bed complement plan)	TBD	Ongoing	
c. Review implementation of pediatric service			
• Support physician recruitment as needed			
• Incorporate facility needs into facility master plan			
• Assess opportunities for pediatric surgical services			
1.4 Other clinical services are identified and significantly enhanced based on market need and opportunity; consider services such as digestive diseases, geriatrics, health and wellness, and others			N. Jones
a. Create a business planning process that identifies all current non-COE programs and services and new program development opportunities	< $25,000	June 2010	
• Assess potential opportunity and vision			
• Assess resource needs			
• Assess financial performance and ROI			
b. Evaluate potential program development initiatives using the business planning process	< $25,000	June 2010	
c. Identify growth, maintain, or divest strategies for each current and potential program or service	< $25,000	Ongoing	

© 2011 Health Strategies & Solutions, Inc.

Often, a senior manager will be assigned primary responsibility for implementation activity related to a specific goal and will assemble an implementation team to work on the goal. Depending on the complexity of the assigned area and scope of implementation activities required, the team may consist of as few as 2 or 3 individuals or as many as 20.

During this final task of the strategic plan development process, each implementation team ordinarily will meet two or three times to flesh out the initial implementation framework. Every organization operates in its own unique manner. Some work best with loose frameworks, similar to Exhibit 6.2, whereas others may significantly expand this chart with additional implementation detail for each action. One important additional consideration increasingly incorporated into these frameworks is a contingency plan for complex, difficult, and risky strategies.

However the organization proceeds, momentum must be maintained. Implementation should begin as rapidly as possible, often before the plan is actually adopted by the organization. It should proceed as envisioned, with appropriate modifications as needed, so that the organization can move toward realizing its vision and goals.

Much more will be said about the important topic of strategy implementation later, but now is an appropriate point at which to introduce it. Most experts concur with Swayne, Duncan, and Ginter (2008): "Implementation is as much a job of strategic leadership as strategy formulation...and effective strategy implementation requires the same determination and effort that is devoted to situation analysis and strategy formulation."

Corboy and O'Corribui (1999) identify the following "seven deadly sins...that doom effective strategy implementation":

1. **The strategy is lacking in terms of rigor, insight, vision, ambition, or practicality.** If the strategy is simply more of the same, comfortable, and incremental it will not create the excitement needed for successful implementation.

2. **People are not sure how the strategy is to be implemented.**
   Leaders are too impatient to make the strategy happen so
   they don't communicate details about how implementation is
   to proceed. They sometimes consider communication time-
   consuming indecisiveness.
3. **The strategy is communicated on a "need to know" basis
   rather than freely throughout the organization.**
4. **Some or all aspects of strategy implementation lack a specific person in charge.** Failure to carefully see to all aspects of
   implementation results in oversights and confusion.
5. **Strategic leaders send mixed signals by dropping out of
   sight when implementation begins.** The absence of strategic
   leadership implies that implementation is not worthy of their
   attention and, therefore, unimportant.
6. **Unforeseen obstacles to implementation occur and responsible people are not prepared to overcome them in creative
   and innovative ways.**
7. **Strategy becomes all consuming and details of day-to-day
   operations are lost or neglected.** Strategy is important but
   so are operations.

ADOPTION OF THE STRATEGIC PLAN

If planning activities have proceeded smoothly up to this point,
adoption of the strategic plan is fairly simple and straightforward.
The steps to formally approve the strategic plan include

- preparation of an executive summary;
- preparation of the strategic plan document;
- resolution by the strategic planning committee recommending
  approval of the plan by the board;
- for hospitals and health systems, review and input by medical
  staff leadership;

- formal and informal educational sessions and presentations of the strategic plan to the board; and
- strategic plan approval by the board.

THE EXECUTIVE SUMMARY

Preparation of an executive summary of the strategic plan is sometimes overlooked in the rush to move from planning to implementation. However, this document is often the only strategic plan output read by many board members and other important stakeholders. When new board members and senior staff members join the organization in the first few years following completion of the strategic plan, the executive summary provides a critical perspective on both the organization and its direction and strategies.

The executive summary (two to three pages in length) should include the rationale for preparation of the strategic plan, background on the planning process used, major findings, and major recommendations. Exhibits 6.4 and 6.5 present sample one-page summaries of major recommendations. Exhibit 6.6 is a two-page summary that illustrates how the strategic plan recommendations align with the pillars of excellence framework, a common performance improvement tool used by many healthcare organizations. Some organizations issue the executive summary as a stand-alone document, with the strategic plan as a separate companion document. Others place the summary in front of the complete strategic plan document.

Whether the executive summary is prepared as a stand-alone document or integrated into the strategic plan, a complete strategic plan document should be prepared at the conclusion of the planning process. The strategic plan document should include the outputs of all planning activities and a description of important process steps (e.g., interviews, retreats). This document serves as the record for all that occurred during the planning process and provides a reference of analyses and supporting information that may be germane to implementation.

Exhibit 6.4: Memorial Hospital Strategy Planning, 2003

MISSION
(Organization's purpose—for internal and external audiences)

Memorial Hospital provides quality healthcare with skill and compassion, meeting the lifelong healthcare needs of all citizens of Smithton and the surrounding communities.

VISION
(What Memorial Hospital aspires to be in five to ten years—for internal audiences)

Memorial Hospital will be the best choice for quality healthcare.

STRATEGY STATEMENT
(Principal method to achieve the vision—primarily for internal audiences)

"Patient centered and performance focused."

GOALS

- Adopt a product line approach to clinical and financial management, which includes a proactive approach to performance improvement.
- Enhance the hospital's image, promote product lines, and increase market share.
- Expand or develop new services and product lines to generate new revenue of $5 million over five years.
- Be an employer of choice and develop a culture of service excellence. Be ranked in the top 5 percent in patient and employee satisfaction.
- Strengthen relationships with physicians.
- Develop local solutions to insurance crisis.

COMMITTEE REVIEW

The complete strategic plan document usually is viewed in draft form by senior management and the strategic planning committee before being finalized. Most organizations provide a copy of the strategic plan document to all board members prior to discussion of approval by the board. The complete document is also distributed to the senior management team. Further distribution of the document

Exhibit 6.5: OHS Strategic Plan Summary 2008

OHS Organizational Direction

Our Health System will be the healthcare leader in the region, providing exceptional medical care and service for every patient, every day, in a patient-centered, family-focused environment.

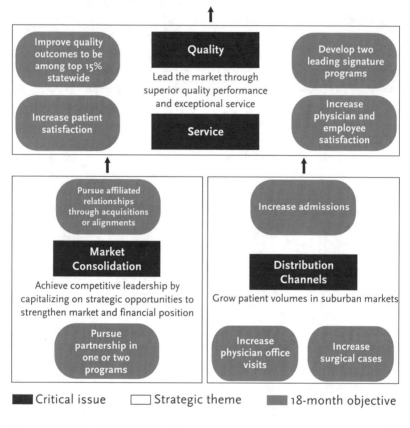

© 2011 Health Strategies & Solutions, Inc.

or the executive summary is discretionary depending on the sensitivity of material included in the report, extent of competition and potential for strategy "leaks," and potential recipients' need to know.

Usually, limited changes in wording or format may be suggested by the committee, with the main purpose of the meeting

FY 2012 Vision and Strategic Issues	People	Quality	Service	Innovation	Growth	Finance
Vision: Clinical excellence	•	•	•	•	•	•
Full leadership commitment to the vision	•	•	•			
Undersized clinical enterprise growth			•			
Clinical focus	•		•	•	•	•
Quality distinction	•	•		•		
Financial improvement					•	•

Pillar of Excellence / with vision statement underneath (continued)

Exhibit 6.6: UCSD Medical Center Strategic Plan Summary 2007; Aligning the 2012 Strategic Plan Vision and Strategic Issues with the Power of Excellence Pillars

FY 2012 Vision and Strategic Issues	People	Quality	Service	Innovation	Growth	Finance
Responsibilities for change at all levels of leadership	●					
Standard faculty compensation plan that aligns pay with performance and rewards clinical excellence	●	●	●			●
Communicate current performance on quality and demonstrate improvement in three areas	●	●				●
Operational changes to achieve three metrics that contribute to clinical excellence across the enterprise	●	●	●			
Leadership and related organizational structure for cardiovascular and cancer	●					
Search for at least one clinical star in each area of emphasis	●	●		●	●	
Invest in and proactively nurture clinical excellence within the organization	●	●	●	●	●	●
Organization-wide behavior standards to improve patient satisfaction scores	●		●			
Clinical availability (appointment slots) for patients to improve payer mix and to reduce wait times for appointments			●		●	●

Source: UCSD Medical Center (2007). Used with permission.

to recommend the plan to the board for approval. Often, this final meeting is also used to discuss next steps and implementation, and to outline how the committee will be involved in subsequent strategic plan updating or implementation monitoring.

In hospitals and health systems that include hospitals as a major component, review of the strategic plan by medical staff leadership is usually a desirable step to take before the board formally considers the plan. Although substantial variation exists in how this step is carried out, some medical staff review and input on the plan is almost always sought by board members.

Medical staff participation in this stage may range from one-on-one or small group consultations with a few carefully selected staff leaders (especially in highly competitive environments) to meetings with the medical executive committee or other medical leadership groups to broader-based input in the most participative environments. The nature of the dialogue with the staff is to seek out fairly high-level input as opposed to more detailed or parochial input, although some of that may be provided anyway. Finally, medical staff approval of the plan is rarely requested, so it is important to reinforce that input, not approval, is being requested.

BOARD APPROVAL

In most healthcare organizations, at least one full presentation of the strategic plan to the board is provided prior to formal review by the board. This educational session, which may be conducted in a retreat format, provides an opportunity for the full board to review and question the plan's analyses, findings, and recommendations. This type of session is intended to increase the board's understanding of the plan and its implications for the organization and to allow any important issues about the plan development process and subsequent implementation to surface and be discussed.

For most healthcare organizations, one educational session of this type is the only major activity required before formal board consideration of the plan. However, some organizations require a second educational session, small group discussions, or one-on-one meetings between board members and the CEO. Senior management and leadership of the strategic planning committee must do whatever is necessary to ensure that board members understand and support the strategic plan. Strategic planning leadership should be especially sensitive to board members' concerns, confusion, or discomfort and attempt to directly address board member needs so that the full board is genuinely enthusiastic about strategic plan adoption and implementation.

The board review and approval process of the strategic plan may encompass a limited number of steps carried out over a few weeks, or a significant number of steps over a few months. This is largely a function of the complexity of the plan, its recommendations, and the organizational style of the hospital, such as the degree of deliberateness in the review and approval process.

Rarely is the strategic plan not approved, though sometimes the board returns it to the planning staff or committee for major rework. If the staff and committee have done their jobs well, including gathering extensive input and communicating with all elements of organization leadership, the board approval process should proceed without any serious roadblocks.

Adoption of the strategic plan by the board should be a mere formality. If this is not the case, either appropriate preparation did not occur or sensitivity to board concerns was lacking.

MONITORING AND UPDATING THE STRATEGIC PLAN

Ongoing Review and Revision

Approval of the strategic plan should not be viewed as the end of planning, but rather as the beginning of the next phase. In today's healthcare delivery environment a comprehensive and thorough strategic planning process should result in a strategic plan that has a useful life of three to five years. The plan will need to be updated or fine-tuned during that period. In fact, strategic planning should be viewed as an ongoing activity of the organization (discussed and described further in Chapter 9). Even in years when a complete plan update is not required, there should be an annual calendar of strategic planning activities, including limited update of the environmental assessment, modification of goals, and preparation of new or revised objectives and actions.

Monitoring progress in achieving strategic plan goals and objectives is especially important; in some cases, goals or objectives are abandoned because they are not achievable or no longer desirable. As a result of implementation activities or strategic plan update analyses, contingency strategies or actions may be deployed, and the primary strategy or action deemphasized or halted.

Every organization should commit to a regular, formal process of tracking and monitoring progress of the strategic plan. In the first year of a plan, many organizations monitor progress monthly or bimonthly. Assuming good progress is being made and significant external or internal changes are not occurring, formal progress tracking and monitoring may be conducted with decreasing frequency later but probably need to occur at least quarterly if the plan is to remain effective.

Often, the strategic planning committee continues in an active role after the strategic plan is completed, overseeing the annual update and monitoring implementation at a high level. An example agenda for the strategic planning committee that operates in this manner is provided in Exhibit 6.7.

Interim-Year Activities

At a minimum, two major planning-related activities should occur in the off years when a comprehensive strategic planning process is not underway: updating and implementing the plan. In some organizations, responsibility for both of these activities is assigned

Exhibit 6.7: Strategic Planning Committee Responsibilities

Regular Meetings (Quarterly)	Annual Strategic Plan Review and Update
I. Review summary progress report (report card, status of objectives targeted for completion since last meeting, etc.) II. Receive detailed update on select objectives*, focusing on variances from metrics or timetable III. Direct appropriate follow-up • Corrective action plans for problem areas • Adjust objective time frames as necessary • Appropriate communication to full board IV. Discuss major new environmental changes and effects as applicable	I. Receive an updated environmental scan from management II. Review entire strategic plan in an expanded strategic planning steering committee session III. Reexamine all goals, objectives, and metrics • Add, modify, or delete as necessary IV. Identify objectives for next year and direct management to prepare necessary action plans and timetables V. Develop strategic plan status report (in partnership with management) to present to the full board

* Select objectives are reviewed in detail at each quarterly meeting; over the course of the year, all objectives are reviewed. Report card data compiled by management.

© 2011 Health Strategies & Solutions, Inc.

to the same party, which can be a group of senior management staff or the strategic planning committee. Even if the responsibilities for carrying out these activities are divided between two groups, the activities need to be linked and communication must occur regularly between the responsible parties.

In those years in which a limited update of the strategic plan occurs, a record of the update process and output (e.g., Strategic

Plan Update for [Year]) should be created to update the full board or formally modify the approved strategic plan. Many healthcare organizations conduct an annual board retreat, which is a good forum for reviewing the year's progress and setting direction for the next year.

STRATEGIC PLAN COMMUNICATIONS AND ROLL OUT

Some organizations do an exceptionally good job of communicating strategic planning results and moving into the implementation phase, while others do not. Why does such wide variation occur?

Few would argue against the importance of communicating the results of strategic planning and making an effective transition from planning to implementation. What appears to be at issue is the degree of formality and the extent of the communications process as well as the rigor and need for structure in transitioning to implementation. Earlier in this chapter, the case for rigor and structure in the implementation process was outlined and the pitfalls of a lack of leadership commitment to implementation were defined. Effective management of the implementation process will be discussed further in Chapter 9.

Another key element of a successful transition from strategic planning to implementation is a strong communications process. Organizations that move smoothly and effectively from planning to implementation communicate broadly and use completion of the strategic plan to signal to key stakeholders that a new era is beginning. The use of celebration as a communications element garners attention and interest and raises expectations.

The communications process should inform and involve constituents. A sample communications plan is presented in Exhibit 6.8. By sharing strategic plan findings, recommendations, implementation priorities, and sequence with key individuals and groups, the prospects for plan acceptance and implementation support are enhanced. An example of a narrative strategic planning summary

Good Tips

Exhibit 6.8: Potential Ideas to Incorporate into Communications Plan

Internal Communications	External Communications
• Communicate directly with frontline employees as often as possible to ensure buy-in of strategic initiatives • Train executives and managers to convey strategic initiatives and core values in a consistent manner • Articulate accountability so that staff members have a clear understanding of responsibilities • Reinforce strategic initiatives through symbolic representation, such as posters or signs • Use multiple networks: town hall meetings, employee newsletters, intranet postings, webcasts/podcasts	• Create summary document for marketing materials and media distribution • Post succinct and clear outline of strategic plan on website • Create presentation with a review of strategic plan for CEO to give to community groups • Schedule appearances before various community constituencies (church groups, chamber of commerce, etc.)

A well-organized communications plan will be an essential part of the strategic plan rollout.

© 2011 Health Strategies & Solutions, Inc.

that may be used during the communications process is included in Appendix 6.1.

Fogg (1994) outlines some of the most important considerations in designing and effectively carrying out a strategic plan communications process. The following are three central aspects of the communications plan:

1. Audiences that need to be addressed:
   - Senior management/boards

- Their subordinates
- Other employees (in most healthcare organizations medical staff members and key external constituencies should be added).

2. What to tell each audience:
   - Tailor information to the jobs and positions of the audience.
   - Take into account the information that they need to carry out their part in the plan.
   - Be sensitive to the group's need to know proprietary information and/or the strategies agreed on.
   - As a general rule, the more people know about the vision and strategic plan, their role in it, and its effect on their job, the better. This knowledge helps direct spontaneous action, plans, and programs at lower levels in the organization. It also reduces working at cross purposes and misunderstandings about what is strategically important (e.g., quality versus cost reductions).

3. The best method of communicating the plan:
   - Develop scripts and visual aids for each major target audience so that a uniform message is conveyed.
   - Have a senior manager, preferably a member of the planning team, present the plan to each target group.
   - Leave time for employees (and others) to ask questions and get answers, preferably in small groups with managers facilitating them and recording issues.

Fogg (1994) also suggests that strategic plan communication is not a one-time event and that consistent effort and attention of the CEO and senior staff are necessary to carry out this communication successfully. While the planning process may be technically complete when the board approves the strategic plan, all of the hard and creative work may be for naught if a sustained effort is not carried through into implementation.

CONCLUSION

This chapter addresses a successful transition from planning to implementation of the strategic plan. A thorough, structured approach to this transition is recommended in five key steps:

1. Assign implementation responsibilities
2. Communicate and roll out the plan
3. Complete additional detailed planning where necessary
4. Set up a system to monitor progress during implementation
5. Commit to regular plan updates

Because the transition from planning to implementation has been especially difficult for many healthcare organizations, a leadership-driven, carefully managed, and clearly articulated approach to this phase is required. As a result, the transition should be accomplished more smoothly and should position healthcare organizations for a higher rate of implementation success.

Strategic Plan Example

ONE MISSION, VISION AND VALUES FOR ALL OF UW HEALTH

MISSION: OUR REASON FOR BEING.

Advancing health without compromise through

- Service
- Scholarship
- Science
- Social Responsibility

The new mission reflects an emphasis not only on excellence in providing care for specific episodes of illness, but also on making individuals and populations healthier overall. We pledge to do that without compromise—that is, always in the best interests of patients and populations and with treatments and programs that provide the right care at the right time by the right person in the right place.

The new mission also contains the four core purposes that have always defined all three UW Health partners. These are expressed as:

- **SERVICE** – providing the best possible patient care experience and outcomes for all those who need our services as well as programs that support the health and wellness of individuals and populations.
- **SCHOLARSHIP** – delivering contemporary education for the current and future generations of health professionals.
- **SCIENCE** – conducting a broad range of research to discover the most promising ways to promote health and to prevent, detect and treat illness in people and in communities.
- **SOCIAL RESPONSIBILITY** – doing what is best for the individuals and communities we serve through policy advocacy, health care delivery and public health.

VISION: OUR PLACE IN THE WORLD.

Working together, UW Health will be a national leader in health care, advancing the well-being of the people of Wisconsin and beyond.

The most important change in the new vision is captured in the first two words, *working together*. These words express the major difference between this strategic plan and all previous ones: The commitment of all three UW Health organizations to work collectively as a single enterprise. The vision also explicitly documents UW Health's commitment to promoting health and our intention to be an even stronger player on the national stage.

VALUES: THE IDEALS WE LIVE BY.

- **EXCELLENCE:** We strive to be the best, and we work continuously to improve our performance and exceed expectations.
- **INNOVATION:** We pride ourselves on finding new and better ways to enhance quality of care and all aspects of our work.
- **COMPASSION:** We treat patients, families, learners and each other with kindness and empathy. We connect with patients and family individually and personally and engage them as partners in decisions about their care.
- **INTEGRITY:** In all our decisions, we are guided by doing the right things at the right time in the right place. We focus on the best interests of patients. We are always honest with each other, learners and our patients.
- **RESPECT:** We honor patients' right to privacy and confidentiality. We value differences among individuals and groups and we actively listen, encourage feedback and choose the best way to deliver timely and meaningful information.
- **ACCOUNTABILITY:** We hold ourselves individually and collectively responsible for the work we do and for the outcome and experience of every patient, every learner, every day.

UW HEALTH STRATEGIC PLAN

UW Health's Five-Year Strategic Plan, 2010-1014, represents a true milestone: The first time all three UW Health partners—UW Hospital and Clinics, UW Medical Foundation and UW School of Medicine and Public Health—have created a single plan with a single mission, vision, values and strategic goals.

Brief background

The development of the plan followed this unified approach. Leaders from all three organizations participated equally in the creation of the plan and are equally committed to achieving its vision. Although the plan formally includes only the clinical departments of UW SMPH, it recognizes that the full academic and educational missions of the school are essential to UW Health's overall commitment to excellence as an academic health center.

The decision to create a single plan was reinforced by interviews and surveys among faculty, staff, administrative leaders and governing boards, as well as patients, families and other stakeholders. Marketplace findings, industry trends and prospects for health care reform also made a compelling case for a unified plan.

UW Health is fortunate to embark on the next five years from a position of solid strength—in the marketplace, in recognized clinical excellence and in financial health. Each organization has developed independently and achieved success on its own. The next five years offer the exciting opportunity to fulfill the promise of our highly regarded brand—harnessing our collective strength to bring unsurpassed patient care and service to the people of Wisconsin and beyond.

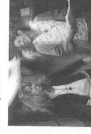

OVERALL STRATEGY AND GOALS

UW Health's overall strategy for the next five years is to provide unsurpassed patient care, harnessing the power of our academic endeavors and a new level of market responsiveness and leadership.

Pursuing this strategy will require us to bring together all the clinical and academic resources of UW Health to meet the needs of patients—not only for routine primary and specialty care but also for the latest in clinical and translational research and the expertise, diverse viewpoints and close attention to care in a teaching and learning organization. The unified strategy will enable UW Health to make nimble decisions and respond quickly to a rapidly changing marketplace.

QUALITY DISTINCTION

Goal

UW Health truly provides outstanding patient care and is clearly distinguished as a quality and patient safety leader in the nation.

Why it Matters

UW Health is already honored with recognition as a national leader in many aspects of quality and safety. By 2015, we are committed to perform consistently across the board in the top decile of health care systems. This goal covers all required and/or publicly reported quality and patient safety measures for both inpatient and outpatient care. Where applicable, it also covers prevention and wellness measures aimed at the health of populations. To support and reinforce this level of quality distinction, UW Health will continue to build and strengthen a culture of safety and continuous improvement.

Five-Year Initiatives

- Establish shared leadership and accountability for quality and patient safety at all levels of UW Health.
- Develop a culture of safety and continuous improvement with high levels of reporting and a non-punitive environment.
- Align physician rewards and recognition with participation in quality/patient safety initiatives.
- Strengthen three to five processes/systems each year that will improve quality and patient safety.
- Make maximal use of research and technology to improve quality and patient safety.

SERVICE EXCELLENCE

Goal

UW Health provides patient-centered care and is clearly distinguished for its culture of service excellence.

Why it Matters

Patient-centered care leads not only to greater patient satisfaction with their health care experience, but also is associated with better outcomes of care. As health care teams help patients and families understand and participate in decisions about their care, they gain valuable insight into patients' health status and life circumstances. This knowledge helps shape plans of care and leads to improved quality. The culture of service excellence also will extend to referral relationships among internal and external physicians and among colleagues in all roles throughout UW Health. These strong collegial relationships will support the ultimate goal of patient-centered care.

Five-Year Initiatives

- Integrate service excellence standards and create a culture of accountability throughout UW Health.
- Upgrade and standardize systems and processes across UW Health to create as seamless a care experience as possible for patients and families.
- Actively engage patients, families, employees, learners and volunteers in pursuit of service excellence in partnership with clinicians, staff and administrators.
- Improve communication with and responsiveness to internal, local, and regional referring physicians.
- Improve timeliness and ease of access for patients.

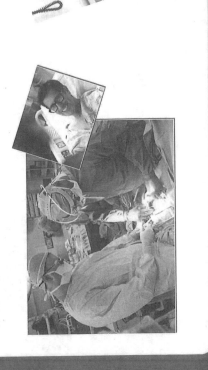

INTEGRATION AND ALIGNMENT

Goal

UW Health functions as though it is a single clinical enterprise.

Why it Matters

Patients and regional partners know UW Health by our among and highly regarded UW Health brand. They rightly expect to receive the same excellent care and service in each and every UW Health clinic or hospital setting they visit. They also expect seamless interactions and hand-offs by caregivers as they move from one care setting to another. This goal requires that by 2015, UW Health will have a seamless set of clinical operations across all settings. Ambulatory care standards will be fully met at all UW Health clinics and both patients and external partners will experience UW Health as a fully integrated clinical enterprise. Wherever possible ambulatory services will be delivered as shared UW Health services. When services are not shared, they will be delivered in such a way that organizational differences will be transparent to patients and other customers.

Five-Year Initiatives

- Develop a UW Health culture that shows commitment to working together and advances the vision of the enterprise and its academic and clinical missions.
- For ambulatory care, create one system for management, governance and operations, with one set of performance standards.
- Expand shared decision making and accountability, including additional joint committees and more shared services across UW Health.
- Modify UWHC service lines, as appropriate, to become UW Health service lines that foster and build on innovations derived from academic endeavors.
- To the fullest extent possible, pursue a UW Health approach to implementing all aspects of the strategic plan.

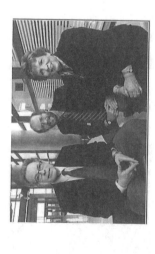

CLINICAL PRIORITIES

Goal

Beginning with three clinical areas, UW Health implements a state-of-the-art, organization-wide model of care that will be recognized for:

- Excellent clinical outcomes
- Innovation
- Academic excellence
- Superior cooperation among roles and disciplines
- High demand and/or market dominance, both locally and regionally.

While the model will be developed initially in three areas, it will eventually encompass existing service lines and other clinical areas.

Why it Matters

To help reach our goal to function as a single clinical enterprise, UW Health will by 2015, develop an organization-wide model of care that ensures excellence, consistency and collaboration across settings. Clinical priorities identified in the plan have been selected based on the readiness and suitability to develop and implement such a model in a particular area. The model will foster not only clinical excellence but academic distinction and faculty recognition. Maintaining and enhancing our role as a national leader, we will be in the vanguard in bringing new clinical technologies and disease/care management processes to market. The effectiveness of the model will be reflected in the process and outcome measures by which UW Health—and the health care industry—evaluates quality, safety and the overall patient experience.

Five-Year Initiatives

- Develop and implement the state-of-the-art, integrated model of care in three initial areas: breast care, digestive diseases and women's health.
- Expand UWHC service lines to span all of UW Health.
- Operate all expanding and newly created service lines within a UW Health framework.

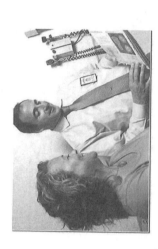

GEOGRAPHIC STRATEGY

Goal

UW Health is the premier provider of subspecialty care in Wisconsin and adjacent portions of bordering states and significantly increases national patient referrals.

Why it Matters

Strong regional and national relationships are essential for UW Health to fulfill its vision to be a state and national leader in health care, advancing the well-being of the people of Wisconsin and beyond.

Achieving this vision will require excellence in tertiary and quaternary services to attract regional and national patients, and geographic outreach that brings UW Health experts to regional communities. We will build and strengthen partnerships with regional hospitals, primary and secondary care physician practices. It will also require the engagement of our local and regional referring physicians through streamlined organizational process improvements and dedicated physician-to-physician relationship building.

Five-Year Initiatives

- Proactively pursue affiliations in select strategic markets, offering a clearly defined continuum of affiliation options while maximizing the value of our existing affiliations.
- Build on current referral and academic relationships, Unity Health Plans and other managed care products, and owned or affiliated primary care practices.
- Enhance communication and services for referring providers.
- Identify and maximize the delivery of programs and services that distinguish UW Health as an academic health center and the premier provider of subspecialty care.
- Capitalize on new technologies and clinical and translational research efforts.

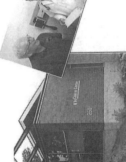

PRIMARY CARE

Goal

UW Health has an advanced primary care model that drives health status improvement in Wisconsin by improving access and fostering appropriate use of health care services and optimal specialty care.

Why it Matters

Primary care is UW Health's "front door" for many patients—a unique milieu in which they first become acquainted with our enterprise and form a medical home from which all of their care is coordinated and managed. These patients seek and deserve easy and timely access to care that is culturally sensitive, quality-driven and makes full use of technologies and educational and community resources. Staff in primary care clinics seek and deserve a sustainable and professionally satisfying environment that supports excellence at all levels. An advanced primary care model therefore will require a culture of quality, service, respect and trust that fully empowers patients; values all members of the health care team and facilitates use of resources to provide the best outcomes and experience for all.

Five-Year Initiatives

- Redesign the primary care model in conjunction with academic partners, evaluating the composition and roles within care teams, care delivery approaches and opportunities to optimize information technology.
- Advance the care of populations with chronic illnesses.
- Include primary care clinics outside Dane County in primary care redesign initiative efforts.
- Support primary care clinics for medical home certification.
- Continue to encourage students to pursue careers in primary care, through residency programs and through efforts such as the Wisconsin Academy of Rural Medicine (WARM) and Training in Urban Medicine and Public Health (Triumph).

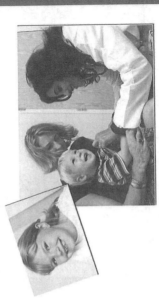

HEALTH CARE'S BEST WORK AND ACADEMIC ENVIRONMENT

Goal

UW Health is health care's best work and academic environment.

Why it Matters

Much of our success over the life of this strategic plan will depend on the ability of UW Health leaders to communicate its vision and on employees' understanding of how to bring that vision to life in their day-to-day roles within the enterprise. Staff and leaders who have this understanding and belief in the organization's mission and goals will be accountable and will commit extra effort to achieve success.

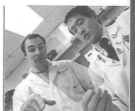

This goal recognizes that investing in leadership and in a healthy, collaborative work culture of engaged staff is important not only for employees but also for health professional trainees. For them, UW Health is a learning laboratory that will set the tone for their entire careers.

Five-Year Initiatives

- Develop and engage the skills and talents of leaders across UW Health through integrated leadership development programs that include standard competencies, 360-degree feedback, leadership orientation on-boarding, talent review, succession planning and developmental assignments across UW Health.
- Develop a process of accountability for all UW Health leaders, faculty and staff with standardized performance expectations, selection criteria, performance review process and methods of recognition and rewards.
- Advance the integration and alignment of human resource management across UW Health through strategies such as:
  o Optimal learning environments for students, employees, trainees and faculty
  o Increased learning and development programs and opportunities
  o Common recognition and retention strategies
  o Integrated employee health services where appropriate
  o Integrated employee/faculty wellness program with health risk assessments
  o Common engagement survey while preserving individual organization's ability to measure and respond to their workforce
  o Integrated appreciation and community service events
  o Uniform employment-related policies
  o Standard structures and guiding principles for select leaders to work across UW Health
  o Common technology infrastructure needed for shared programs
  o Common recruitment efforts to provide staff to fulfill the mission and vision

CHAPTER 7

Major Planning Process Considerations

It is good to have an end to journey toward, but it is the
journey that matters most in the end.

—*Ursula K. LeGuin*

The most important things a leader can bring to a changing
organization are passion, conviction, and confidence in
others. Too often executives announce a plan, launch a task
force, and then simply hope that people find the answers—
instead of offering a dream, stretching their horizons, and
encouraging people to do the same. That is why we say,
'leaders go first. . .'

—*Rosabeth Moss Kanter*

Nearly all experts agree that structuring and carrying out an effective strategic planning process is more important to the organization and the success of strategic planning than the strategic plan
itself. The increasing complexity of the healthcare environment
and the growing vulnerability of healthcare organizations to environmental and competitive threats have made it far more challenging to come up with effective strategic plans.

At the same time, the increasing size of healthcare organizations
and the diversity and complexity of many of these organizations,
especially the large multi-entity systems, has significantly increased
communications difficulties and rendered these unwieldy organizations difficult to manage. While it is possible to overdo the strategic planning process and derail or overwhelm the organization's
capacities, in general more process is better than less. As a rule,

organizations should strive to maximize participation in the planning process within the limits of their capabilities to handle it and achieve the desired results.

Key to an effective planning process is developing shared understanding and, ultimately, consensus about four important elements of the strategic plan:

1. Environment, including current and especially future
2. Critical issues the organization faces
3. Mission and vision to guide the organization to the future
4. Major plan outputs, including priority strategies and alternatives considered

An effective process builds acceptance, facilitates approval, and expedites the transition from planning to action.

The planning process needs to link effectively the many constituencies involved in healthcare organizations. If it does so, it can facilitate better communication among staff and improved coherence in future operations. While the organization should certainly seek tangible outputs from strategic planning, the planning process presents important opportunities for improving communication across the organization, and forging new and stronger bonds among stakeholder individuals and groups to help ensure the organization's future viability.

This chapter addresses some of the critical elements of the planning process. While many of these elements have been mentioned in passing in previous chapters, the importance of a strong planning process calls for more extended discussion.

FACILITATION

An extremely critical element of a successful strategic planning process is the facilitation. Someone needs to be primarily responsible for guiding the process throughout, ensuring that the important planning tasks are conducted and completed, assisting leadership and other key groups involved in the process to reach decisions and achieve consensus, and then directing the transition from planning to successful implementation. While many individuals involved in the strategic planning process will have specific responsibility for facilitating one or two aspects of the diverse group work, one person typically takes the lead throughout, with overriding responsibilities for the entire process.

What alternatives exist for effective facilitation support of the strategic planning process? Many healthcare organizations have a planning staff or organizational development department (or occasionally other internal resources) that can facilitate the planning process. Some organizations retain consultants to fill this role. When evaluating possible consultants, organizations should look for individuals who are highly experienced, have industry and comparable organization experience, and possess a range of facilitation skills described further below.

In some instances, the CEO may consider serving as the process facilitator. Most CEOs will find this an extremely challenging job to carry out well, if for no other reason than it makes productive group discussion and consensus development difficult. Most CEOs inhibit free discussion due to their power and authority and tend to dominate meetings when put in charge. Avoid this alternative if at all possible.

Fogg (1994) suggests that the best facilitators have three types of skills (see Exhibit 7-1):

- **Process**: Putting the planning process together and making it work
- **Content**: Giving specific solutions to business and strategic problems
- **Intervention**: Breaking personal, organization, and business decision blockages

Exhibit 7.1: Facilitator's Job Description

What the Facilitator Does

I. PROCESS

- Structure
  - Structures the process
  - Defines key analyses
  - Produces the manual
  - Handles documentation
- Training
  - Trains in planning and process
- Facilitation
  - Facilitates major meetings
  - Teaches others to facilitate
  - Gives private advice on process
  - Schedules meetings
- Resourcing
  - Identifies training
  - Identifies outside facilitators
  - Identifies content specialists

II. CONTENT

- Solutions to specific strategic issues

III. INTERVENTION

- Diagnostic interviewing
  - Initial
  - In process
- Private counsel, particularly CEO
- Team interventions
- Keeps process on time

What the Facilitator Does Not Do

- Develop the plan
- Write the plan
- Make decisions
- Become a power point
- Play politics
- Execute the plan

When the Boss Facilitates; Is Part of the Team

- Be a member of the group
- Speak last
- Use good facilitator skills
- Be neutral
- Let the team come to consensus
- Do not dominate or be authoritarian
- You always have the deciding vote—use it sparingly

Source: Fogg (1994), p. 46. Used with permission.

He adds that all three types of skills may not be, and often are not, possessed by any single individual. The more of the three skills that are offered by one person or group, the more effective and efficient the strategic planning process will be. In nearly every strategic planning effort, all three types of skills are needed and the organization must be prepared to provide them at appropriate points in the process. Fogg believes that the lead facilitator must have certain basic process skills, especially a keen understanding of all parts of the planning and implementation process and how to weave them together successfully, knowledge of organizational behavior and the change process, and strong leadership capabilities.

TEAMWORK

Much of the strategic planning process occurs through the efforts of informally or formally constituted diverse groups. In the typical strategic planning process, important teamwork will occur through the strategic planning committee, board of trustees, senior management staff, and a variety of standing or ad hoc groups. How can the effectiveness of these many and varied groups be maximized?

Fogg (1994, 257) suggests that effective teams are "characterized by:

- Considerable discussion
- Open communication
- Debate, even conflict, on key issues
- Decision by consensus whenever possible
- Monitoring, measuring, and correcting of their own team behaviors"

Effective teams must also have a clear charge or objective to accomplish, good leadership by a chair who facilitates and directs but does not dominate, and accountability of the team and individual members for results. Among other qualities, individual team members must be good listeners, constructive participants, and willing to put aside their own self-interest for the sake of the group. All

Exhibit 7.2: Team Interventions

Process
- Facilitate team mission; roles, job description, and processes used
- Process checks during and at end of meetings—what is good and bad versus norms
- Redirect process when off track
- Point out dysfunctional team behavior

Meeting
- Off agenda or subject—get team back on track
- Summarize or crystallize key points; transitions
- Offer stand-up facilitation when team is bogged down
- Crystallize, facilitate, and resolve conflicts
- Missing the point—suggest it

Content
- Wrong decision—point out correct options or process to define correct decision
- Suggest expert outsiders
- Give specific content solutions

Individual
- Point out dysfunctional individual behavior or interactions
- Offer individual or pair counseling

Source: Fogg (1994), p. 52. Used with permission.

in all, a very tall order, but one that is essential to the smooth and successful flow of activities in the strategic planning process.

The interaction of the facilitator(s) and team is a critical element of an effective strategic planning process. Fogg (1994) provides a useful checklist (Exhibit 7.2) of facilitation tips to keep the teams on track and moving ahead.

PLANNING RETREATS

Almost every strategic planning process will have at least one planning retreat. The retreat will usually bring together board members, physicians, and other clinicians and management in an extended planning session. Some retreats are intended for board members exclusively, while others are for members of different leadership groups. Depending on the organization's style and preferences, as well as the particular focus of the retreat, the retreat may be held off site and may even be carried out in a remote location and combined with social and recreational activities. A review of the purposes of the different types of retreats that may be held during the strategic planning process is presented below.

Kickoff Retreat

Some organizations use a retreat at the beginning of strategic planning to jump-start the process and create enthusiasm and momentum. The agenda for this type of retreat may include some or all of the following:

- Rationale for strategic planning (purpose and expected benefits)
- Strategic planning orientation (per Chapter 2)
- Review of previous planning efforts, successes, and failures
- Review of the organization's recent performance
- Discussion of the organization's strengths, weaknesses, opportunities, and threats (SWOT)
- Review of current major strategic initiatives
- Identification on a preliminary basis of major planning issues

Often, one or more outside keynote speakers will be used to discuss critical issues or environmental challenges. This type of retreat is a good vehicle for underscoring the importance of strategic planning and creating heightened interest in the planning process from the outset.

Midprocess Retreat

At any number of points in the middle of the strategic planning process, retreats can be held to

- focus on a particular issue of concern;
- have extended discussion that is not possible within a regular planning committee session;
- obtain broad-based input, including the members of the planning committee and other important leaders not represented on the committee; or
- brainstorm about approaches to issues facing the organization.

External speakers may be used in midprocess retreats in a manner similar to kickoff retreats. The purposes of a midprocess retreat are information sharing, clarification, and direction. These retreats are rarely used for decision making or communicating "answers" to strategic planning issues at this stage in the process.

Concluding Retreat

At or near the end of the strategic planning process, a retreat may be held to

- obtain additional, broad-based input before finalizing the recommendations;
- communicate the answers (i.e., what the plan's key recommendations are);
- serve as a bridge to implementation, including strategizing about implementation opportunities and barriers; and
- build a broader consensus on the plan and its recommendations than that represented within the planning committee alone.

Often, this type of retreat will be developed to expose all members of the board to the strategic plan before it is brought to this group for formal consideration of its adoption. This type of retreat may also be used to signal the organization that planning is (temporarily) over and implementation is about to begin.

Retreats may be held in off years, when a full strategic planning effort is not undertaken, to accomplish any of the purposes cited above, and to keep the planning process going even as the organization's efforts are primarily devoted to implementation. Increasingly, healthcare organizations are holding one or two planning retreats per year to review and revise the strategic plan, make important corrections to the direction and strategies, and obtain broad-based consensus on key initiatives to keep the organization moving forward. These retreats are an excellent vehicle to maintain planning momentum and organizational commitment in the face of day-to-day pressures that consume management and have the potential to take the organization off course.

RESEARCH APPROACHES

Much of the success of the strategic planning process is dependent on information gathering and involvement of key constituencies, which come through various research efforts. The importance of constructive involvement of key constituencies in the strategic planning process cannot be overstated; implementation is dependent on a broad base of support for the plan's recommendations and actions. This support is only likely to occur if stakeholders believe they have a true opportunity to shape the results. A brief review of the range of research approaches used in strategic planning follows.

Interviews

Interviewing is typically part of every strategic planning process. Individual or group interviews usually occur early in the strategic planning process to gather information and demonstrate sensitivity to the perspectives of internal parties, but also to accomplish one or both of these purposes with external parties. Occasionally, interviews may be carried out during the middle of the process to gather additional information on issues of concern or involve select parties in review of alternative approaches for addressing particular issues.

Surveys

Surveys are the second most frequently employed technique and they are often used for information gathering early in the strategic planning process. Many organizations participate in ongoing survey efforts that provide valuable input for strategic planning—patient satisfaction, quality/outcomes tracking, and consumer perception are among the most common. Surveys may be carried out internally to gather broad input in a less expensive way than is possible through other research approaches. Internal surveys may also allow each member of an affected group to be involved in the strategic planning process, and to accomplish this participation in an equitable and consistent manner. External surveys have similar purposes. The advantages and disadvantages of different survey approaches—electronic, mail, or telephone—as information-gathering techniques are best left to experts in this subject area (see, for example *Designing and Conducting Survey Research: A Comprehensive Guide* by Rea and Parker). With the availability and prevalence of electronic communication today and various standard survey tools, such as SurveyMonkey, much focused surveying is occurring via the Internet or organizational intranets.

Focus Groups

The focus group technique is the least frequently used of the three approaches, but is growing more common in strategic planning processes. Focus groups may be convened at any point in the process to gather information on a particular issue. Such groups are becoming a popular activity in the strategy formulation stage of the planning process and provide excellent forums for multidisciplinary development of strategy on a given issue. The advantages and disadvantages of focus groups versus other research approaches is a larger subject than can be addressed here (see, for example, Stewart, Shamdasani, and Rook 2007).

A modified version of a focus group is the reactor panel. Depending on the substance of the material to which a reaction is being sought, reactor panel members may be key constituents of a particular group (e.g., cardiovascular providers) or more diverse in representation (e.g., the medical executive committee). When conducting a reactor panel during the strategic planning process, the facilitator is usually seeking a focused response to a particular recommendation, set of recommendations, or potential alternatives under consideration. Reactor panels are appropriate vehicles for these narrowly defined purposes.

Most strategic planning processes employ more than one of the above approaches. With the growing recognition of the importance of a strong process in strategic planning, more extensive use of individual and group research approaches in strategic planning can be expected and should be encouraged in future planning efforts.

KEY STAKEHOLDER INVOLVEMENT

The strategic planning process is more likely to succeed if all key stakeholders understand their roles. A brief description of each major group's roles follows.

Board Members

The strategic planning committee is usually an ad hoc or standing committee of the board and therefore includes significant representation from the board of directors. Board members will be important participants in retreats and involved in internal research. The board should be concerned with the policy implications of strategic planning and is generally and appropriately focused on the organizational direction portion of the strategic planning output.

Physicians

In hospitals, health systems, and, obviously, medical groups, physicians should be well represented on the strategic planning committee. They will often be the group that is the subject of the most extensive research of the internal (and sometimes external) constituencies.

Physicians should be concerned with the clinical implications of strategic planning; in teaching hospitals and academic medical centers they will also be concerned about teaching and research interrelationships with clinical services and specific recommendations affecting the academic role of their organizations. Physicians may be most broadly affected by the outputs of the strategic planning process, but except in some of the second or later generation integrated delivery systems, they do not have direct approval authority or clear implementation responsibility.

Few topics are as hotly debated today as how to involve medical staff members in hospital and health system strategic planning. The escalation of competition between physicians and hospitals over provision of outpatient services and, increasingly, entire high-margin clinical service lines, has created enormous complexity and confusion in this area. Recently, with more physicians being employed by hospitals and health systems, this dynamic is changing. Further change may occur as this trend continues and healthcare reform spurs more significant integration.

While no single approach fits every situation, constructive and careful physician involvement in the planning process is vital to effective planning. Appropriate accommodations will need to be made for competitive considerations in many instances. Little or no involvement of physicians in strategic planning is not an option.

Senior Management

Senior management is almost always represented on the strategic planning committee, but generally in smaller number and "voice" than board members or physicians. Management, however, plays an important and central role as the coordinator of the strategic planning process—structuring the process, staffing it, keeping it moving along, and overseeing implementation. Senior management's role and responsibilities in the planning process generally increase as it reaches its later stages.

Other Clinicians

Depending on the nature of the organization, other clinicians (e.g., nurses, physical therapists, psychologists) may play a major or minor role in the strategic planning process. In healthcare organizations not dominated by hospitals or physicians, other clinicians may have significant involvement, including participation on the strategic planning committee of the board. In hospital- or physician-dominated healthcare organizations, other clinicians will play a minimal role or have no role in the strategic planning process but will usually get involved when implementation begins or is near.

Other Management

In most cases, other management members will only get involved in the strategic planning process prior to implementation if a significant issue or area of concern arises over which they have direct responsibility or expertise. Although some strategic planning experts advocate a bottom-up strategic planning process that calls for broad-based and extensive participation from all levels of the organization, few healthcare organizations practice such an approach (as discussed further below). A summary of the typical involvement of key stakeholder groups in major elements of the planning process appears as Exhibit 7.3.

While every planning process is carried out somewhat differently, Exhibit 7.3 summarizes the sections above and can be used as an initial framework for structuring involvement at the outset of strategic planning. It may be reconsidered as the process moves along.

ADVANCING PROCESS TO THE NEXT LEVEL: EMPHASIZE BOTTOM-UP VERSUS TOP-DOWN STRATEGIC PLANNING

Strategic planning in healthcare is still very much a top-down process. Dominated by senior management (see Exhibit 7.4), and to some degree, the board, planning in most organizations engenders little participation, awareness, and ultimately support from the majority of employees, and even less from customers. Strategic planning in large healthcare organizations is still very hierarchical, with business units and other subsidiary entities reacting and responding to edicts and directives from on high.

Practices in leading firms outside of healthcare are almost exactly the opposite. While corporate leadership provides high-level direction and guidance, planning is increasingly focused in

Exhibit 7.3: Typical Involvement of Key Stakeholder Groups

	Approval	Steering Committee	Interviews/ Research	Retreats	Strategy Development	Implementation
Entire board	✓			✓		Oversight
Planning committee of the board	✓	✓	✓	✓	✓	Oversight
Physicians		✓	✓	✓	✓	✓
Senior management	✓	✓	✓	✓	✓	✓
Other clinicians			✓			✓
Other management			✓			✓
Planning staff	←———————— Support entire process ————————→					

© 2011 Health Strategies & Solutions, Inc.

Exhibit 7.4: Participation of Stakeholders in Healthcare Strategic Planning

	1 No Participation	2 Limited Participation	3 Moderate Participation	4 Considerable Participation	5 Extensive Participation	N/A Unsure	Mean Response
Board members	5% (20)	20% (78)	27% (103)	26% (101)	18% (69)	3% (13)	3.33
Physicians	3% (12)	19% (72)	35% (133)	30% (113)	12% (46)	1% (5)	3.29
Other clinicians	9% (35)	35% (131)	33% (124)	17% (63)	4% (14)	2% (9)	2.70
Senior management	0% (1)	2% (9)	7% (26)	26% (99)	64% (247)	0% (1)	4.52
Middle management	5% (19)	21% (82)	38% (146)	29% (111)	6% (22)	1% (3)	3.09
Outside community leaders	31% (119)	39% (148)	18% (70)	8% (30)	1% (5)	3% (10)	2.07
Outside customers/ patients	38% (147)	39% (149)	14% (55)	4% (15)	1% (3)	3% (13)	1.86
					Total Respondents		384

© 2011 Health Strategies & Solutions, Inc.

the business units or other subsidiary parts of the company and driven up, rather than down, the organization.

This approach has many benefits: it allows broader-based, more substantial, and more meaningful participation in the planning process; generally encourages creativity and innovation; has the "real action" of planning taking place closer to the customer; facilitates organizational support for what results from the planning process; and leads to greater implementation success. In addition to senior management providing vision and direction and championing the process, such organizations must have a culture of trust and accountability, outstanding formal and informal communication networks, and sound strategic skills across the organization.

A decentralized planning process is much harder to manage than a centralized one, and, of course, such a process risks loss of control. However, leading companies have found that the benefits of a decentralized process far outweigh the negatives and that it delivers much more overall value. Some healthcare organizations are beginning to move in this direction, but as an industry, much progress is needed to approach this best practice outside of healthcare.

ADVANCING PROCESS TO THE NEXT LEVEL: USE AN EVOLVING, FLEXIBLE, AND CONTINUOUSLY IMPROVING PROCESS

Even today, too many healthcare organizations are wedded to a process that has worked well historically and are reluctant to make significant changes. "Why fix what isn't broken?" some ask. While there is value and security in the tried and true, regular advances in approaches and methods are occurring in strategic planning in healthcare and outside of it. Therefore, aspects of a process that is five or ten years old—or even one year old—may not be current enough to keep the organization in the forefront. Executives certainly aren't content with yesterday's operations management or financial planning and management approaches, so why shouldn't strategic processes be evolving, too?

The quality and continuous improvement orientation of an organization's strategic planning process can be evaluated by examining the process at three increasingly challenging levels of inquiry.

First and most basic, is the current process comprehensive, objective, timely, and highly participatory throughout the organization?

Second, does the process link effectively to operations and to individual and group performance objectives in the organization?

Third, does the process include continuous learning so that process deficiencies are identified and corrected before the next planning cycle begins?

Organizations with flexible, continuously improving planning processes are able to adapt more readily to the changing environment that is characteristic of healthcare today. These organizations employ planning processes that are far more externally oriented than the typical healthcare organization. They use external factors and forces to create the platform for change that is necessary to keep strategic planning alive and vital.

CONCLUSION

This chapter illustrates that the use of an effective strategic planning process is at least as important to organizational success as the actual plan itself. When structured and carried out with care, the facilitation, planning retreats, research, and involvement of key stakeholders can lead to a highly successful planning process that maximizes participation and secures a commitment to plan implementation.

SUGGESTED READINGS

Rea, L. M. and R. A. Parker. 2005. *Designing and Conducting Survey Research: A Comprehensive Guide*. San Francisco: Jossey-Bass.

Stewart, D. W., Shamdasani, P. N., and D. Rook. 2007 *Focus Groups: Theory and Practice*. Thousand Oaks, CA: Sage Publications, Inc.

CHAPTER 8

Realizing Benefits
from Strategic Planning

In a period of upheaval, such as the one we are living in,
change is the norm. To be sure, it is painful and risky, and
above all, it requires a great deal of very hard work. But
unless an organization sees that its task is to *lead* change,
that organization—whether a business, a university, or a
hospital—will not survive.

—*Peter F. Drucker*

The true measure of your worth includes all the benefits
others have gained from your success.

—*Cullen Hightower*

Why should an organization carry out strategic planning? What
benefits can be expected from this effort? How can the strategic
planning process be structured and managed to maximize the likelihood that the benefits will be realized? These and other related
important questions will be addressed in this chapter.

Unfortunately, while the case for strategic planning may seem
obvious, strategic plans regularly fail to achieve their promise.
And the enactment of healthcare reform in 2010 should materially
increase the drive to achieve benefits, particularly in topic areas
historically neglected by strategic planners and plans.

Survey results in healthcare and non-healthcare literature reveal
that many organizations struggle with realizing the benefits of
strategic planning. Bruton, Oviatt, and Kallas-Bruton (1995) conducted an extensive survey of the literature on this subject and

found little conclusive evidence of the benefits of strategic planning. They cite some non-healthcare studies that suggest that service firms that carried out strategic planning performed worse than those that did no planning. They also reviewed 12 empirical studies, conducted over the previous 20 years, of the effectiveness of strategic planning in hospitals. That review shows decidedly mixed results.

Similarly, in a strategic planning survey of healthcare executives conducted by this author in 2005 to 2006, benefits realization was not judged to be at the same level as the quality of the plans developed and planning processes (Zuckerman 2007). Respondents perceived that despite effective strategic planning processes, strong plans, and reasonably good implementation, the results achieved (i.e., benefits) did not meet expectations.

The author's experience over the past 35 years suggests that these findings are related to the failure of leadership to (1) clearly state at the outset of strategic planning what benefits should be achieved through the process, and (2) keep benefits realization on the front burner throughout the process and then into implementation.

Some organizations plunge into strategic planning without ever identifying what may be gained through the process. Others state so many expected outcomes that it is difficult to interpret or remember what the main purposes are, whereas others provide only vague expectations so stakeholders are not really sure what strategic planning's purpose is. Still others get off to a clear, good start, but then veer off course during the process through inadequate, inconsistent, or contradictory communications about intended benefits.

IDENTIFYING STRATEGIC PLANNING BENEFITS

This chapter will discuss the substantive (i.e., non-process related) strategic planning benefits that can be identified at the outset and pursued throughout the process. These benefits should fall into one or more of four categories:

1. Product and market improvement
2. Financial improvement
3. Operational improvement
4. Community needs realization

The following sections review each category of benefit and describe what is desirable and possible to achieve.

Product and Market Improvement

Historically, strategic planning has been oriented toward achieving product and market benefits. Larger service areas, higher market shares, more comprehensive products and services, and, recently, improved linkages among services have formed the core of healthcare strategic planning's concerns. Relative to other areas of potential benefits, product and market improvement has been addressed fairly well by healthcare organizations.

Exhibit 8.1 presents an illustration of the most prevalent outcomes historically versus the desired planning impact for each subcategory.

- **Market (service) area**. Every healthcare strategic plan is at least somewhat focused on protection, if not expansion, of the market or service area of the organization. Even in the most rural areas and certainly in all urban and suburban areas, the geographical area primarily served by the organization is at least partly of interest to competing providers and increasingly under significant competitive attack. Because of the growing competitive nature of healthcare, offensive strategies that target new geographical markets are quite common. Despite the primacy of this topic area, strategic planning efforts have achieved mixed results with their attempts to grow or defend service areas.

Exhibit 8.1: What Product or Market Benefits Can and Should Be Achieved?

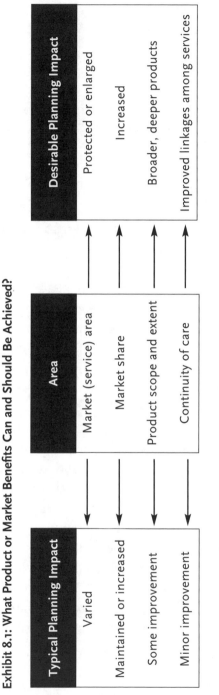

Typical Planning Impact	Area	Desirable Planning Impact
Varied	Market (service) area	Protected or enlarged
Maintained or increased	Market share	Increased
Some improvement	Product scope and extent	Broader, deeper products
Minor improvement	Continuity of care	Improved linkages among services

© 2011 Health Strategies & Solutions, Inc.

- **Market share.** Equally prevalent are strategies to increase existing market shares. Most strategic plans conclude that market share increases are necessary and feasible. And in the majority of cases such conclusions and strategies do lead to increased shares.
- **Product scope and extent**. A growing number of healthcare organizations are recognizing that growth of products (i.e., programs and services) can no longer be handled in an unsystematic manner, but needs to be explicitly addressed and managed. As a result, an increasing proportion of strategic plans deal with this issue directly by recommending broadening the product mix, deepening the offerings of existing products, or both. Attempting to formally manage product scope and extent is a fairly recent issue for healthcare organizations; strategic planning results are moderately positive to date.
- **Continuity of care**. An even newer issue—basically a second-generation consequence of integrated delivery—is attempts to strengthen continuity of care through the strategic planning process. While most organizations that remain committed to vertical integration recognize that benefits realization depends on improved linkages among services, these benefits have proven difficult to achieve. Leaders have begun to appreciate that achieving such benefits in integrated delivery systems takes time and thus continuity of care is an increasingly important strategic planning topic.

FINANCIAL BENEFITS

This category of likely substantive benefit is probably the most obvious and is applicable to all healthcare organizations; however, benefits realization has been, at best, mixed in this category.

Exhibit 8.2 identifies four general areas of financial improvement benefit along with the historically most prevalent outcome versus the desired planning impact.

Exhibit 8.2: What Financial Benefits Can and Should Be Achieved?

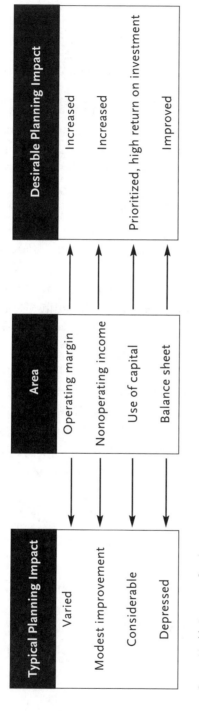

Typical Planning Impact	Area	Desirable Planning Impact
Varied	Operating margin	Increased
Modest improvement	Nonoperating income	Increased
Considerable	Use of capital	Prioritized, high return on investment
Depressed	Balance sheet	Improved

© 2011 Health Strategies & Solutions, Inc.

- **Operating margin.** Few, if any, healthcare organizations have such a high operating margin that they can ignore the need to maintain or increase it. For many organizations today, increasing the operating margin is the primary goal of strategic planning. Unfortunately, too often plans are developed to "meet community needs" or satisfy internal constituents without appropriate regard for the impact on operating margin and the financial position generally. As a result, and consistent with the results of the literature on strategic planning, plans are just as likely to decrease operating margin as they are to increase it.
- **Nonoperating income.** This issue has not been a high-priority topic for many healthcare organizations until fairly recently. The bull market of the 1990s and the bear market of the early twenty-first century, however, has raised the profile of this issue considerably. In addition to sound investment management, an increasing number of healthcare organizations have targeted philanthropy as a high-priority strategy. Such organizations have developed sophisticated, comprehensive fundraising programs and generate significant nonoperating income for use in capital projects, as seed money for clinical program investment, and to build endowments. A small number of organizations have developed large-scale clinical research enterprises, consulting practices, and other nonpatient care ventures to tap into nonoperating income sources. However, the lessons of the 1980s suggest that diversification away from the core healthcare business can be difficult and should be approached cautiously.
- **Use of capital.** Another typical reason for commencing strategic planning is to help structure or rationalize capital-intensive facilities and technology development investments. Strategic planning is commonly used outside of healthcare for the purpose of making difficult choices among alternative capital and operating investment decisions. A small but growing number of healthcare organizations use the strategic planning process in a similar manner, which, in turn, should result in a ranking

of potential capital projects according to return on investment, both financial and nonfinancial. Unfortunately, even today, some strategic plans lead to capital consumption without appropriate regard for the downstream financial impact.

- **Balance sheet.** Only rarely, despite the increasingly difficult financial climate in healthcare, is improvement of the balance sheet stated as a desired strategic planning outcome. And, given the discussion above, it is understandable that the balance sheet can often deteriorate as a result of strategic planning. Nevertheless, few organizations today can afford to see their balance sheets suffer, even if that suffering results from important projects being carried out. Balance sheet management has not been a priority in the planning process among nonfinancially oriented executives and trustees in healthcare organizations, but it needs to be much more of a concern in the future.

Case Example

Catholic Health System (fictitious name) is a large integrated delivery system, with 2010 revenues of about $1 billion. Operating in a metropolitan area, the system had been in severe financial distress, resulting in the replacement of the chief executive officer early in 2007. The new CEO initiated a strategic planning process in the latter part of 2007, with the main goal of across-the-board financial improvement.

The results of the strategic planning process are impressive. Operating margin increased from negative 1 percent in 2007 to 6 percent in 2010, primarily as a result of strategic pricing increases, growth of high-yield services, focus on high margin outpatient growth, and operational improvements, particularly in regard to managed care contracting and productivity.

The organization initiated a formal development program for the first time in its history, which resulted in completion of a $20 million capital campaign and commencement of annual giving and bequests components. A major accomplishment was achieved in the area of capital prioritization: In 2007, capital requests and needs through 2012 were estimated to be nearly $600 million (a considerable amount of catch-up deferred capital spending was on the table); the strategic planning process eliminated certain projects and trimmed back others so that the capital budget was reduced to $400 million. With improvement across the balance sheet toward an A-rated system underway by 2011, capital needs can be financed without significant negative effects on the balance sheet.

OPERATIONAL BENEFITS

In contrast to financial benefits, the operational benefits category is probably the least recognized category of potential strategic planning benefit. Yet, it is applicable to nearly all healthcare organizations, and tremendous potential may be realized in operational improvement through strategic planning. Many aspects of this category will increase in strategic importance over the next decade.

Exhibit 8.3 identifies four general areas of operational improvement benefits, along with the historically most prevalent outcome versus the desired planning impact.

- **Patient satisfaction**. In a service industry such as healthcare, few topics are as important to success as satisfied customers. Yet, customer satisfaction was not a major concern of healthcare organizations until the relatively new competitive era emerged in the 1990s, brought on by managed care and resulting excess supply and financial difficulties. Now, with the increasing availability of information comparing healthcare organizations to each other, customer satisfaction has moved from the background to the foreground in competitive and, therefore, strategic importance. Plans that do not acknowledge

Exhibit 8.3: What Operational Benefits Can and Should Be Achieved?

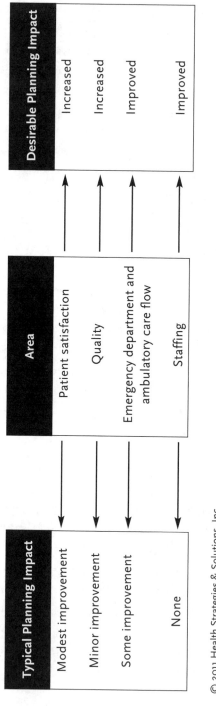

Typical Planning Impact	Area	Desirable Planning Impact
Modest improvement	Patient satisfaction	Increased
Minor improvement	Quality	Increased
Some improvement	Emergency department and ambulatory care flow	Improved
None	Staffing	Improved

© 2011 Health Strategies & Solutions, Inc.

or, better yet, address this factor, are likely to fall short of the mark in terms of critical benefits realization.

- **Quality.** Much as customer satisfaction was a major concern of the general public, but not providers, until about ten years ago, quality was in a similar position until the late 1990s. With the publication of the Institute of Medicine's report *To Err is Human* (1999), the problem of safety in healthcare organizations, and quality generally, came out of the closet. The first efforts to measure and publicize healthcare quality across like organizations now are taking hold. The availability of comparable data on quality makes quality improvement a strategic imperative in the coming years. Tremendous gains in quality are likely to emerge, and strategic plans need to move beyond the traditional measures of volume and financial improvement in clinical programs to accommodate and influence the critical developments in quality.

- **Emergency department and ambulatory care flow**. The majority of healthcare consumers access services in an outpatient setting, yet hospitals and health systems are still primarily oriented to an inpatient-dominated business. Nearly all organizations have Byzantine and difficult operational processes that consumers face when they access emergency and other outpatient services. Because of the magnitude of problems in this area, its large and growing importance as a centerpiece of state and national reform initiatives, and the capital and incremental operating expenditures required to address these issues, this topic has hit the radar screen of some strategic planners in the past few years, with modest success to date and much more needed in the future.

- **Staffing.** Growing shortages of nursing and certain allied health personnel have become one of the most widely acknowledged problems and threats to the success of healthcare organizations. Despite the significance of this issue, it is on the strategic agenda of only a handful of organizations; others expect the human resources department and various operational executives to deal with this situation out of sight of strategic planners and the strategic planning process. The magnitude of the problem, its systemic nature, its likely long-term duration, and its extension into some physician specialties are causing the staffing shortage to become an important strategic topic. The result of this attention should be some strategically driven interventions and improvements in the coming years.

Case Example

Regional Hospital and Health System (RHHS; fictitious name) is a medium-sized hospital and diversified healthcare organization, with 2010 revenues of about $180 million. Operating in a small metropolitan area, RHHS competes with larger, financially stronger hospitals and systems, all of which have the resources to outspend and outflank most traditional strategic initiatives that RHHS undertakes.

RHHS's CEO determined that the organization's advantages in service and processes represented competitive advantages that could be leveraged more strategically. Accordingly, the 2005 and 2009 strategic plan updates focused on maximizing the benefits that could be obtained in these areas.

The results of the strategic planning efforts are especially impressive given the lack of interest and progress in customer service issues experienced throughout the industry to date. RHHS implemented a highly tailored, innovative customer service program and brought its patient satisfaction scores up from the top 25 percent of its peer group nationally in 2005 to the top 10 percent by 2008, and the score was nearing the top 5 percent by 2010. RHHS was the first hospital in its region and state to successfully pursue magnet status designation from the American Nurses Credentialling Center, gaining this recognition in 2006.

RHHS implemented a state-of-the-art emergency department redesign in both facilities and operations between 2008 and 2010, bringing online dedicated urgent care services and chest pain, stroke, and observation care programs. It used its magnet designation, strategic compensation program, and exemplary staff satisfaction and patient care environment to achieve tremendous success in staff recruitment and retention, resulting in the lowest attrition and vacancy rates in the region. All of its efforts have led to continued healthy volume growth each year for the past five years, solid financial performance, and an extremely positive environment and reputation for RHHS in its region.

COMMUNITY BENEFITS

Traditionally, not-for-profit healthcare organizations have attempted to derive and demonstrate community benefits from their strategic planning. Often, however, this area of benefit is "talked up" more than it is actually addressed. Not-for-profits need to be responsive to the communities they serve. However, as healthcare organizations have grown into larger, more complex businesses, often as part of expansive healthcare systems that operate in many communities (and in some instances states), they have grown distant and detached from the communities that originally spawned them. These large organizations have been unusually preoccupied with internal issues since the integration spurt of the 1990s, further separating them from community concerns and issues.

Exhibit 8.4 identifies four general areas of community benefits along with the historically most prevalent outcome versus the desired planning impact.

- **Needed services provided.** In strategic planning for healthcare organizations, providing needed services was the primary concern for many years and remains an appropriate and important focus today. Providing needed services is probably

Exhibit 8.4: What Community Benefits Can and Should Be Achieved?

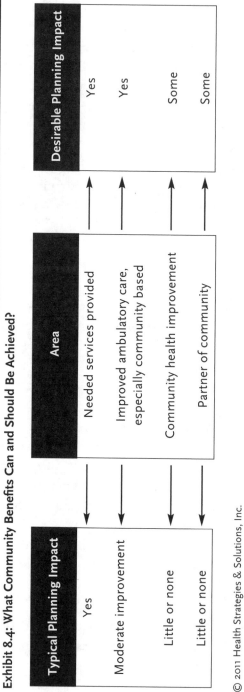

Typical Planning Impact	Area	Desirable Planning Impact
Yes	Needed services provided	Yes
Moderate improvement	Improved ambulatory care, especially community based	Yes
Little or none	Community health improvement	Some
Little or none	Partner of community	Some

© 2011 Health Strategies & Solutions, Inc.

the area of benefit that healthcare organizations address most completely and best. All organizations recognize the importance of structuring service offerings that meet the needs of the constituents they are trying to serve. And healthcare provider competition has traditionally focused on service breadth, depth, and unique or appealing features, thus heightening the importance of this area.

- **Improved ambulatory care, especially community based**. As noted in the previous section, the increasing prevalence of ambulatory care use has made improving its delivery a key competitive concern and important strategic battleground. The growth in ambulatory care demands, the increasing ability of organizations to deliver ever more complex services in community-based settings, and consumer lifestyles and preferences have been a boon to ambulatory care center development since the early 1990s. In many instances, hospitals and systems have strategically led this movement, whereas in others (even within the same organization), it has been met with resistance due to competing priorities and cost and control issues.

- **Community health improvement.** Many healthcare organizations have made community health improvement the centerpiece of their mission statement. Periodically, this area is actually an acknowledged strategic concern of organizations. More frequently, it is given lip service and addressed, if at all, indirectly. Especially for not-for-profits, contributing to community health improvement should be important and a key area of community benefit. Difficulties in demonstrating progress and the conflict of a business that is primarily oriented to treating illness episodically hinder constructive efforts in this area.

- **Partner of community.** All not-for-profit healthcare organizations collaborate with their communities to some degree. As healthcare has become a bigger and bigger business, many organizations have moved away from community partnering. While the challenge of carrying out the typical healthcare organization's mission of "effective caring" in an increasingly complex world might argue for more and better interrelationships with the vast array of community agencies and groups that could contribute to this end, the opposite has occurred; organizations have retreated to primarily doing what they can control (through ownership and operation). While strategic alliances are growing outside of healthcare as a way to address complex situations and issues, they are underutilized as a healthcare resource.

Case Example

Independent Catholic Hospital (ICH; fictitious name) is a relatively small community hospital, with 2010 revenues of about $125 million, operating in a large metropolitan area. ICH has numerous competitors, including many large hospitals, healthcare systems, and university medical centers. ICH is located in a densely populated, somewhat poorer-than-average city neighborhood. The neighborhood has traditionally been Catholic and, while the population has changed dramatically in the past 10 to 15 years, it is still predominately Catholic, albeit with residents of Latin American rather than European origin.

ICH directly and forcefully addressed the topic of community benefits through its strategic planning process in 2008. It reached out to the community through focus groups to better understand the new residents' issues and needs. ICH involved community residents in the strategic planning committee and in task forces formed to address specific issues. The organization subsequently implemented a broad and aggressive outreach program, especially involving the churches, to engage and include the community in the growth and development of the hospital.

Through these and related efforts, the strategic plan identified and targeted high-priority community health issues such as hypertension, stroke, and prenatal care for subsequent action. The hospital determined it needed to rebuild its core services of emergency care, cardiology, and women's health to meet community needs. Furthermore, ICH began a multiyear effort to redesign ambulatory care, particularly to resolve operational and patient access problems, for both on- and off-site services. By 2010, ICH's volumes were slowly climbing and, even more important, its image and reputational scores had advanced considerably over the baseline levels determined at the outset of the 2008 strategic planning process.

CONCLUSION

Strategic planning must become more outcome oriented. Good process is, and will, remain important, but tangible benefits, not just a "feel good" ending, need to be achieved. Deriving benefits starts with identifying and communicating categories and types of benefits that could be realized through strategic planning at the outset of the process.

Four different types of substantive benefit—product or market, financial, operational, and community—and 16 subcategories of possible benefits within these broad categories have been reviewed in this chapter. Leadership needs to agree which benefits should be realized through the strategic planning effort, and the process needs to keep these potential benefits highly visible and continually drive toward their realization. The orientation to benefits realization will make future strategic planning more relevant and effective and help lead strategic planning into a new era of prominence as an accepted and important management discipline in healthcare organizations.

CHAPTER 9

Making Planning Stick: From Implementation to Managing Strategically

Execution is the great unaddressed issue of the business world today. Its absence is the single biggest obstacle to success and the cause of most of the disappointments that are mistakenly attributed to other causes.

—Larry Bossidy and Ram Charan

Ideas are easy. It's the execution of ideas that really separates the sheep from the goats.

—Sue Grafton

Strategic planning has been criticized for its detachment from day-to-day operations and its inability to effect significant change in an organization. While comprehensive, well-designed plans may be prepared with exceptionally strong supporting documentation and the use of thorough, inclusive, consensus development processes, implementation seems to be elusive and ultimately out of reach for many organizations.

Implementation difficulties are not confined to healthcare organizations. According to Mankins and Steele (2005), companies worldwide "typically realize only about 60 percent of their strategies' potential value because of deficits and breakdowns in planning and execution" (see Exhibit 9.1). The Balanced Scorecard Collaborative estimates that 90 percent of all companies fail to execute their strategies (see Exhibit 9.2). A 2005 to 2006 study

Exhibit 9.1: Where the Performance Goes

This chart shows the average performance loss implied by the importance ratings that managers in our survey gave to specific breakdowns in the planning and execution process.

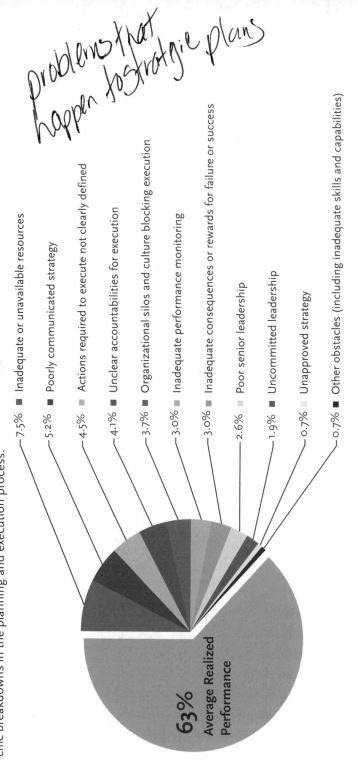

- 7.5% ■ Inadequate or unavailable resources
- 5.2% ■ Poorly communicated strategy
- 4.5% ■ Actions required to execute not clearly defined
- 4.1% ■ Unclear accountabilities for execution
- 3.7% ■ Organizational silos and culture blocking execution
- 3.0% ■ Inadequate performance monitoring
- 3.0% ■ Inadequate consequences or rewards for failure or success
- 2.6% ■ Poor senior leadership
- 1.9% ■ Uncommitted leadership
- 0.7% ■ Unapproved strategy
- 0.7% ■ Other obstacles (including inadequate skills and capabilities)

63%
Average Realized
Performance

Source: Mankins and Steele (2005). Used with permission.

Exhibit 9.2: Four Barriers to Strategy Execution

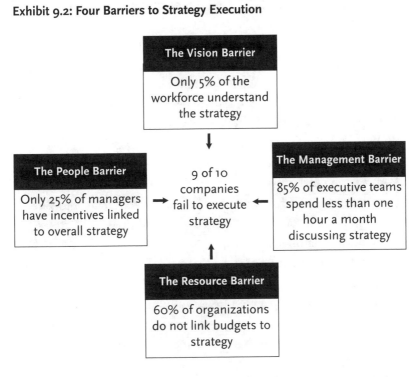

Source: *Balanced Scorecard Step-by-Step: Maximizing Performance and Maintaining Results*, 2nd Edition, by Paul R. Niven. Copyright © 2006 John Wiley & Sons, Inc. Reprinted with permission of John Wiley & Sons, Inc.

of the state of the art in healthcare strategic planning found that effectiveness of strategic plan implementation was rated relatively low by respondents and the ability to handle curve balls and other new developments and adjust the plan and implementation was rated the lowest of all strategic planning skills and components (Zuckerman 2007).

Why is there such a high failure rate in the transition from planning to implementation? It appears to be a function of four main factors:

1. **Loss of energy and focus.** In many organizations, strategic planning is an event that engages a broad spectrum of leader-

ship. It is a high-level, high-visibility process that garners considerable attention and effort. Once the strategic plan has been completed and approved, the show is over and implementation occurs in a much less public and celebrated manner. This loss of energy and focus may ultimately cause implementation to be inconsistent and slowly dissipate over time.

2. **Lack of management.** As described further below, implementation needs to be actively managed. It does not just happen, but requires a significant amount of hard work, direction, and oversight. Yet, in the aftermath of many strategic planning efforts, implementation is assumed to occur rather than be actively managed; in these cases, the implementation failure rate is high.

3. **Disconnect from operations.** Strategic planning is often viewed as an add-on to day-to-day operations; if done periodically, rather than in an ongoing manner, the fragmentation is aggravated. In these situations, the implementation plan does not belong to anyone and is not a part of anything that routinely occurs in operations. This disconnect makes it difficult to maintain a focus on implementation and regularly and consistently make progress.

4. **Lack of resources.** Many strategic plans are overly ambitious and unrealistic. They call for too many activities and actions to be implemented concurrently and devise strategies that exceed the organization's resources. Frustration emerges as it becomes clear that implementation is in jeopardy.

This chapter describes methods and processes to achieve a higher rate of implementation success; integrate strategic planning better into regular, ongoing organizational management; and ultimately evolve from the periodic strategic planning processes of the last 10 to 20 years to the more effective and contemporary strategic management processes of the twenty-first century.

ENSURING SUCCESS IN IMPLEMENTATION

Making a smooth, effective, and ultimately successful transition from planning to implementation starts with a sound, well-understood implementation plan. There is a tendency to rush into implementation at the conclusion of the strategic planning process and not prepare thorough, thoughtful implementation plans. In addition to preparing quality implementation plans, the roles and responsibilities of staff must be understood and accepted, as well as the time frame and interrelationships of implementation activities. Finally and possibly foremost, a management structure and approach to implementation need to be in place. The structure and approach must include, at a minimum, a designated overall implementation leader and regular progress reviews. These reviews could involve senior management, corporate staff (in a system), and/or the strategic planning committee of the board.

As discussed in this author's article, "Executing Your Strategic Plan" (Zuckerman 2005), there are nine steps to successful plan implementation.

1. **Understand that plan execution starts during the preplanning.** The tone, content and approach of an organization's strategic planning process all influence the likelihood of its success. Involve key stakeholders—board members, board planning committee members, physicians, other clinicians, senior and other managers, and planning staff. Communicate the importance of the strategic planning process: Make sure that everyone understands the benefits—community, financial, product/market and operational—of a well-executed plan.

2. **Consider execution while formulating strategy.** Execution is not something to worry about later; it must be an underlying theme during strategy formulation. However, execution worries should not dampen the creative spirit of strategy for-

mulation. Instead, execution issues must be one of the many "planning" and "doing" considerations that occur later in strategic planning. Think about whether high-level strategies can be subdivided into and executed at the operational level. You should be able to align individual actions with organizational strategies.

3. **Choose execution leaders wisely.** Having the right leaders with the right skills in place during plan execution can be the difference between success and failure. When you are selecting execution leaders, carefully consider skill level, ability to engender a sense of strategy ownership, and capacity for communicating. Ensure that leaders have the tools, resources, and training they need. More important, give them the time to finish the job—a chief complaint among execution leaders is a shortage of time. Last, make sure that leaders can resist the urge to meddle. When execution committees are managing implementation well, leaders need to know when to get out of the way.

4. **Mark the implementation phase in a formal, celebratory way.** As planning concludes and execution begins, organizations should select a formal approach for communicating to their staff that implementation is beginning. Assign specific implementation activities, and discuss any further analysis (financial, architectural, etc.) that needs to be conducted. Most important, plan an inclusive roll-out event to show that the planning is complete and a new era is beginning. A celebratory occasion can help draw attention, raise expectations, and build enthusiasm that will be needed during implementation.

5. **Drive the plan down into the organization.** Strategy execution is most successful when it is seen as an organizationwide effort rather than an executive office exercise. Individuals throughout the organization must be given clear directions about what they are expected to achieve. Build implementation tasks into performance objectives and give rewards when they are completed. Using implementation subcommittees—

with no more than 12 members—may help. Consider having these subcommittees in place during the strategic planning process, then transitioning them to a new role in implementation. All organizations may also need to provide training to individuals responsible for implementation.

6. **Watch out for the warning signs of execution failure.** Some common red flags that implementation is not progressing as it should include: persistent political infighting, a loss of focus, a sense of inertia, pervasive resistance to change, and a disconnect between planning objectives and operational realities. If any of these issues crop up, quickly defuse the situation and aggressively pursue getting implementation back on track.

7. **Communicate, communicate, communicate.** Strategy execution involves even more people than strategy formulation, making communication crucial. Establish a common message about the strategic plan, make copies of the plan available, and provide Web-based updates and internal communications via e-mail and other organizational media. Last, the CEO and other senior managers should meet with physicians and staff directly to provide feedback and respond to concerns.

8. **Have a monitoring system in place.** To track the implementation schedule, budget, and progress, use a monitoring system your organization finds relevant, accurate, and useful. Consider using a system that also measures the intangibles—management effectiveness, innovation, and potential for further progress. A good monitoring system will help you review the progress of the plan's implementation. The review should help organizations ensure that progress is being made, priorities stay on track, obstacles to progress are resolved, and resources are reallocated, if needed.

9. **Consider moving from strategic planning to strategic management.** Strategic planning is criticized for its detachment from day-to-day operations and its inability to produce real, sustainable change in organizations. Many organizations use strategic *management* approaches to integrate core management

processes. Strategic management, discussed further later in this chapter, has clear benefits, such as integration (rather than coordination) with finance and operations and the fact that day-to-day management occurs within a strategic framework rather than in separate management processes. Organizations that use strategic management often find that their organizational culture starts adapting to change more easily.

ONGOING REVIEW OF PROGRESS

Fogg (1994) suggests that ongoing review of progress "help[s] you keep the plan on track once implementation is under way, reallocate resources as you accomplish goals or your strategic situation changes, imbed accountability for program accomplishment with every implementer, and reward results to ensure commitment and continued top level performance." He believes that the key to success in this is:

> Review, review, review.
> Revise, revise, revise.
> Reward, reward, reward.

There are five main reasons for conducting regular progress reviews:

1. To shine the spotlight on the ongoing importance of implementation to the organization's success
2. To encourage and motivate individuals and teams involved in implementing action plans through visibility, recognition, and praise
3. To make sure that appropriate progress is being made and that priorities stay on track

4. To discuss and resolve problems and internal obstacles to progress, particularly those that require interdisciplinary intervention
5. To allow reallocation of valuable resources to the areas that most need them

Both formal and informal mechanisms can be used to effectively review ongoing progress. Regular meetings of senior management or the strategic planning committee of the board are one common approach to this task. For many organizations, monthly progress review meetings for the first year or two after completion of a major strategic planning effort help ensure progress and accountability. Frequent progress review meetings are the best way to ensure that implementation occurs and that timely adjustments are made to individual action plans.

Once the organization has accepted a disciplined approach to implementation, less frequent meetings may be required. Mature strategic planning organizations find that quarterly, or, in some instances, semiannual progress review meetings are sufficient to keep implementation on track.

A structured approach to implementation progress reviews often yields the best results. Such structure involves taking action plan formats, such as those provided in Chapter 6, and marking them up in advance of each meeting, charting expectations versus actual results, schedules, resource consumption, and so on. (See Exhibit 9.3). Many organizations use a red, yellow, and green light schema to facilitate review of progress versus plan at a glance. Explanations of variances from expectations should be provided. New issues or concerns, or those that transcend individual action plans, can be noted in a comments section. Recommendations for changes to the implementation plan should also be noted. These progress reports should be circulated to all progress meeting attendees in advance.

Key to making these meetings effective is a structured approach to meeting conduct. An important consideration here is allowing

Exhibit 9.3: Action Plan Progress Review Example: Memorial Health System, Facilities Development Action Plan 9/09

Annual Goals & Measures of Success and Tactics	Resource Requirements	Target Completion Date	Coordinating Individuals	Progress Review				Comments/ Assumptions
				Q1 FY09	Q2 FY09	Q3 FY09	Q4 FY09	
Five-Year Goal and Measures of Success: (2014)								
MHS executes board-approved master facility plan in Lincoln, Springfield, and Taylorville while maintaining a maximum average debt service ratio of 4.5 and days cash on hand of 225								
FY09 Goals and Measures of Success								
SP Objective 11 Execute FY09 components of facility strategy while exceeding maximum average debt service ratio of 3.9 and days cash on hand of 219.								Doug Rahn
a. Obtain approvals and begin construction of ALMH replacement project	High	**9/30/09**	Dalpoas w/ Senior Leadership	GREEN	GREEN	√ 5/2009		CON approved 1/27/09; May groundbreaking
b. Obtain CON and project approval for TMH outpatient services building expansion	Moderate	**9/30/09**	Raab/Johnson w/ Senior Leadership	GREEN	GREEN	GREEN	√ 9/2009	CON approved 9/1/09
c. Obtain board approval for MMC Master Facility Plan	Moderate	**9/30/09**	Rahn w/ Senior Leadership	YELLOW	YELLOW	√ 6/2009		June update to MHS Board SP&D Comm.
d. Complete business and financial planning and formulate recommendation regarding components to be included in phase one of MMC Master Facility Plan	Moderate to High	**9/30/09**	Rahn/Kay	YELLOW	YELLOW	GREEN		Assistance secured to help create a 5-year capital plan
e. Complete plan for reassignment of Koke Mill Medical Center space vacated by OCI	Minimal	**9/30/09**	Rahn w/ Facility Planning Committee	GREEN	GREEN	√ 6/2009		MPS identified as top priority
f. Move CIHOC into Baylis Building	Moderate	**9/30/09**	England	GREEN	√ 3/2009	√ 3/2009		
g. Begin construction of replacement MMC MD parking ramp	High	**9/30/09**	Rahn w/ Facility Planning Committee	GREEN	GREEN	GREEN		Architect retained; city approvals secured

Progress Review Legend: √ Complete (date) = Date completed
GREEN = In progress/on schedule
YELLOW = Caution/potential problem or delay
RED = Decision to stop /major problem

* The resources required are categorized as:
Minimal = 0–25 person days and/or <$50,000 per year
Moderate = 25–50 person days and/or $50,000–$250,000 per year
High = 50+ person days and/or >$250,000 per year

Source: Memorial Health System (2009). Used with permission.

enough dialogue to occur about those action plans and issues that require group attention while minimizing discussion about things that do not require group discussion. In the absence of such focus, progress review meetings tend to be overly long and have diminished effectiveness as a result. In other cases, the meetings are too short and perfunctory.

The meeting leader needs to carefully craft the agenda to balance competing concerns and needs, all within a time frame that is appropriate to the importance of the topics being discussed. Advance preparation and awareness of pitfalls in this process help ensure that the progress review meetings achieve the intended outcomes and are a highly effective mechanism for ongoing plan implementation support.

Individual performance reviews also can enhance the effectiveness of plan implementation. If the action plan objectives are built into individual performance objectives, these annual or semiannual reviews provide an opportunity to review progress and make adjustments with individuals responsible for implementation.

Finally, informal progress reviews can and should occur on an ongoing basis. Contact among senior leadership, some of whom may have direct implementation responsibilities, and between senior leadership and other staff with implementation responsibilities, should be frequent in most organizations. Such regular contact provides yet another opportunity for periodic, but less formal, review of progress against plan.

Even with the active monitoring process outlined above, senior management may need to intervene directly in implementation to keep initiatives on track. Fogg (1994) notes four types of interventions that may be required:

1. Counseling an individual or team, providing advice for dealing with problems or problematic team members
2. Exerting influence to remove obstacles or obtain the resources needed to move forward

3. Improving skills, such as through training or by enhancing functional expertise
4. Providing direction, especially to get an individual or group back on track

Rewards also play an important role in facilitating achievement of implementation tasks. Individual and group performance may both be rewarded, and rewards can be both financial and non-financial in nature. Psychological rewards, including recognition, publicity, and contests, can play a key role in motivating individuals and teams to make good progress in implementation.

THE BALANCED SCORECARD

The balanced scorecard is a tool to assist with ongoing progress monitoring and implementation. Developed in industry in the early 1990s by Robert Kaplan and David Norton, it is intended to supplement traditional performance measurement systems by tracking "financial results while simultaneously monitoring progress in building the capabilities and acquiring the intangible assets [organizations] would need for future growth" (Kaplan and Norton 1996).

The balanced scorecard complements financial measurements with measurements of progress in three key areas: customer satisfaction, internal business processes, and learning and growth (see Exhibit 9.4). Improvements in the balanced scorecard approach have rendered it a valuable tool for some companies that have used it as a key part of a strategic management system (see next section). Kaplan and Norton (1996) suggest that, "used this way, the scorecard addresses a serious deficiency in traditional management systems: their inability to link a company's long-term strategy with its short-term actions."

A number of healthcare organizations have adopted the balanced scorecard as an aid in strategy implementation. Inamdar (2002) cites five potential benefits of this approach for healthcare organizations:

Exhibit 9.4: Translating Vision and Strategy: Four Perspectives

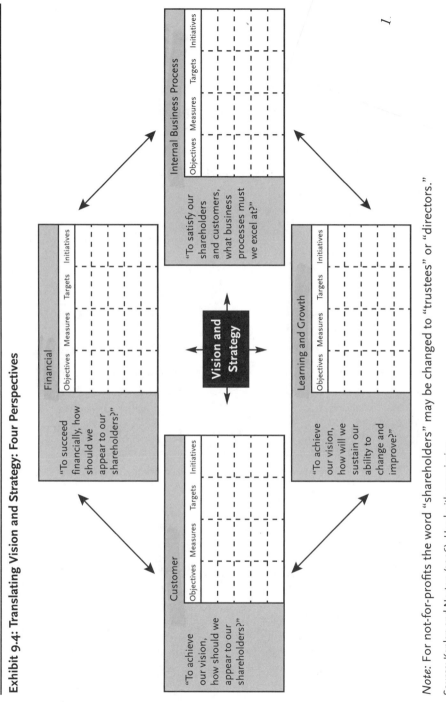

Note: For not-for-profits the word "shareholders" may be changed to "trustees" or "directors."

Source: Kaplan and Norton (1996). Used with permission.

It aligns the organization around a more market-oriented, customer-focused strategy.

2. It facilitates, monitors, and assesses the implementation of the strategy.
3. It provides a communication and collaboration mechanism.
4. It assigns accountability for performance at all levels of the organization.
5. It provides continual feedback on the strategy and promotes adjustments in response to marketplace and regulatory changes.

What is the balanced scorecard? How does it work? Griffith and Alexander (2002) describe it as

an integrated set of measures, driven by the organization's vision and strategy, typically covering the following dimensions in healthcare organizations:

- Financial—financial performance and management of resources (including intangible resources such as workforce capability and supplier relations);
- Internal business processes—cost, quality, efficiency, and other characteristics of goods or services;
- Customer—measures of satisfaction, market share, and competitive position; and
- Learning and growth—measures of the ability to respond to changes in technology, customer attitudes, and economic environment.

In a review of the application of the balanced scorecard approach to healthcare organizations, Inamdar (2002) charted the steps involved in developing and implementing the balanced scorecard (see Exhibit 9.5). Kaplan and Norton (1996) suggest that the process of managing strategy via the balanced scorecard consists of four sequential steps (see Exhibit 9.6):

Exhibit 9.5: The Balanced Scorecard Development and Implementation Process

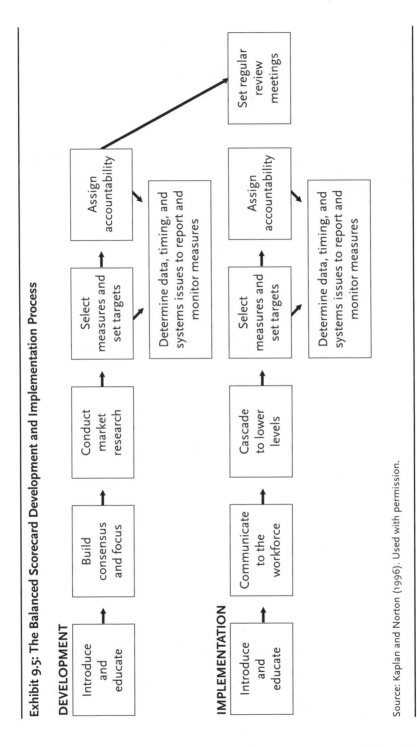

Source: Kaplan and Norton (1996). Used with permission.

Exhibit 9.6: Managing Strategy: Four Processes

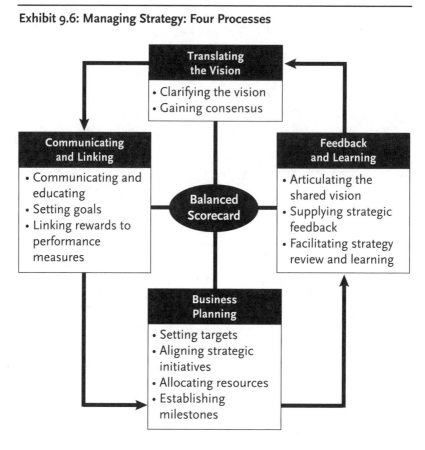

Source: Kaplan and Norton (1996). Used with permission.

1. **Translating the vision.** The mission and vision are often too abstract to be useful to employees as effective guides to day-to-day operations. Identifying concrete measures related to the mission and vision translates these lofty statements into a form that makes them more effective.

2. **Communicating and linking.** Involving employees from all levels of the organization in developing the scorecard initiates the process of integrating it into the organization. Ultimately, linking the scorecard measures to subgroup and individual performance measurement is the most effective approach.

3. **Business planning.** Here is where the overall strategy is translated into the objectives, measures, targets, and initiatives that link the strategy with operations and implementation. Similarly, integration of strategic and budgeting/financial planning is inherent in creation of the scorecard.
4. **Feedback and learning.** A balanced scorecard incorporates a process for review and evaluation of progress and modification of plans as necessary.

While using the balanced scorecard approach improves upon previous performance measurement approaches, Kaplan and Norton (1996) argue that it is even more valuable "as the foundation of an integrated and iterative strategic management system." In these situations, companies are using the scorecard to

- clarify and update strategy,
- communicate strategy throughout the company,
- align unit and individual goals with the strategy,
- link strategic objectives to long-term targets and annual budgets,
- identify and align strategic initiatives, and
- conduct periodic performance reviews to learn about and improve strategy.

FROM STRATEGIC PLANNING TO STRATEGIC MANAGEMENT

Increasingly, healthcare organizations are moving beyond periodic strategic planning to more systematic approaches carried out regularly rather than infrequently and integrated with other core management processes (see Exhibit 9.7). Clear benefits may be derived in implementation rigor and implementation success from ongoing strategic planning and strategic management. Also, the quality of strategic planning and implementation is improved as a

Exhibit 9.7: Transitioning The Strategic Planning Process to Strategic Management

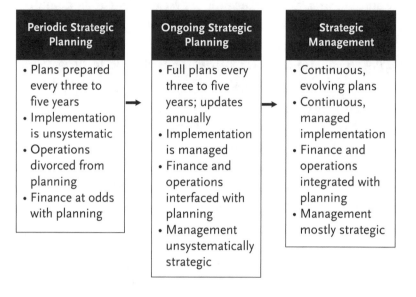

Periodic Strategic Planning	Ongoing Strategic Planning	Strategic Management
• Plans prepared every three to five years • Implementation is unsystematic • Operations divorced from planning • Finance at odds with planning	• Full plans every three to five years; updates annually • Implementation is managed • Finance and operations interfaced with planning • Management unsystematically strategic	• Continuous, evolving plans • Continuous, managed implementation • Finance and operations integrated with planning • Management mostly strategic

result of better coordination with finance and operations in ongoing strategic planning processes. Additional benefits are obtained by those organizations that evolve to strategic management and integrate (versus coordinate) finances and operations with strategic planning as part of their regular management routines. Further, in strategic management, day-to-day management is carried out within a largely strategic framework, rather than the traditional separate strategic management processes for operations, finance, and planning.

What exactly is strategic management? According to Wells (1996), it is

- a systems approach to identifying and making necessary changes and measuring an organization's performance as it moves toward its vision, and

- a management system that links strategic planning and decision making with the day-to-day business of operational management.

Wells (1996) believes that planning is the prelude to strategic management. Strategic planning is insufficient if not followed by the development and implementation of the plan and evaluation of the plan in action.

The balanced scorecard is one proven approach to strategic management. Exhibit 9.8 presents another approach used by healthcare organizations. This approach is a logical extension of a strong strategic planning process transitioning into strategic management. Annually, three concurrent activities take place:

1. The strategic plan is developed or, following a comprehensive strategic planning process, updated in subsequent years. The plan update typically occurs in the first half of the fiscal year. In the second half of the year, planning initiatives provide inputs to capital and operating budgets and plans, and an iterative process leads to the finalization of all budgets and plans.
2. Throughout the year, implementation of the previously developed strategic plan occurs. This is a managed process with ongoing support and oversight of implementation, including formal review of progress and adjustment of implementation as needed. Based on these reviews, implementation of contingency plans for certain initiatives may be required.
3. Operations proceed routinely throughout the year. The implementation is managed within regular management structures and processes and new strategic opportunities are reviewed and tested (with great frequency in some organizations) against the strategic plan. Such reviews may dictate adjustment of the plan's strategies and actions to accommodate new, emerging initiatives.

Exhibit 9.8: Annual Strategic Management Process Components

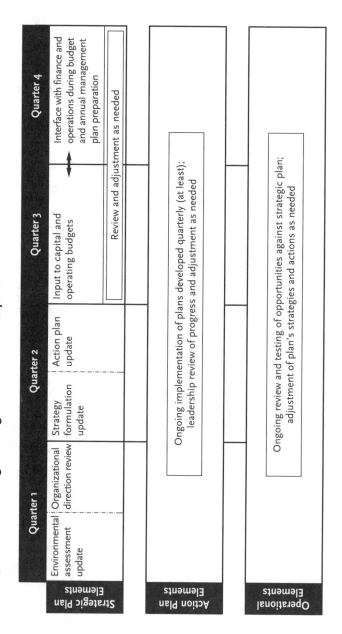

	Quarter 1	Quarter 2		Quarter 3	Quarter 4
Strategic Plan Elements	Environmental assessment update	Organizational direction review	Strategy formulation update · Action plan update	Input to capital and operating budgets	Interface with finance and operations during budget and annual management plan preparation
				Review and adjustment as needed	
Action Plan Elements	Ongoing implementation of plans developed quarterly (at least); leadership review of progress and adjustment as needed				
Operational Elements	Ongoing review and testing of opportunities against strategic plan; adjustment of plan's strategies and actions as needed				

© 2011 Health Strategies & Solutions, Inc.

Whatever process is employed, strategic management represents a powerful tool with substantial benefits for both a stronger strategic planning function and a more successful implementation and integrated operations management function.

CONCLUSION

Effective implementation has proven to be difficult for most organizations. A common misperception is that implementation just happens, when in fact it must be carefully managed if the organization is going to meet its goals and objectives. Ongoing review of progress and new approaches, such as the balanced scorecard, should help keep implementation on track.

CHAPTER 10

The Annual Strategic Plan Update

Reasonable people adapt themselves to the world.
Unreasonable people attempt to adapt the world to
themselves.

—George Bernard Shaw

Greatness is not in where we stand, but in what direction
we are moving. We must sail sometimes with the wind and
sometimes against it—but sail we must and not drift, nor lie
at anchor.

—Oliver Wendell Holmes

As many healthcare organizations move to more of a continuous strategic planning orientation, questions about the scope and extent of the annual strategic plan update arise. Typically, for a few years after a comprehensive strategic planning process has been completed, a far less extensive annual update is required. Fogg (1994) suggests that, on average, it should require one-quarter of the effort of the first plan. But what is the minimum necessary amount of analysis and process, and what might dictate more than the minimum effort?

Despite their professed commitment to an ongoing strategic planning process, some healthcare organizations postpone or permanently put off following through on this commitment. The press of daily operations and operational difficulties can easily delay or derail strategic planning. How can a continuous strategic planning process be hardwired into the organization to limit the risk of things getting off track and strategic planning being relegated to the back burner?

Some healthcare organizations' annual strategic planning processes are robust but not time intensive. How do these organizations invigorate the annual strategic planning effort and leverage its value? Others have done a particularly good job of integrating strategic planning with operational and financial planning. What distinguishes those organizations that have more advanced, integrated processes from the large majority of others that do not? These and other important questions will be addressed in this chapter and should enable healthcare organizations to carry out strategic plan updates more effectively and with better results.

FOCUSING THE ANNUAL UPDATE

As in the full strategic planning process, the annual update benefits from a preplanning stage (per Chapter 2) to focus the quantitative and qualitative work that will follow. Although probably less extensive than the process called for earlier in this book as a prelude to the full strategic planning process, the following, at a minimum, should be determined and communicated before the annual update begins:

- What are the desired outcomes of this strategic planning process?
- What are the key elements of the proposed process and schedule?
- What will be the roles and responsibilities of leaders and groups?
- How will the update be led and organized?

A formal kick-off to the strategic planning process is beneficial to signal that the process is about to begin and to help structure the effort that will follow. A leadership group meeting, written or electronic communication, or some combination of both is a good way to ensure that the update gets off to a strong start.

In most cases the desired outcomes for the annual update follow naturally from the previous planning cycle. Typically, these outcomes involve reviewing and revising the key planning issues and approaches to these issues. In the absence of significant environmental change or organizational difficulties, broadening and deepening the organization's understanding of and approaches to the key issues and making modest midcourse corrections are sufficient to justify continued strategic planning effort.

When significant environmental changes occur, plan implementation is not proceeding well, or the organization is experiencing a crisis (usually financial, but also leadership turmoil and change), a routine annual update process is unlikely to be effective. The desired outcomes in these cases are generally far more extensive and fine-tuning activities will prove to be insufficient.

ENVIRONMENTAL ASSESSMENT

A review of environmental conditions and forecasts is an important part of the annual update. Assuming there are no major changes in external or internal conditions and prospects, Fogg (1994) suggests that the assessment be "surgically updated." That is, rather than updating the whole plan, only those aspects of the plan that have been affected by some change are reviewed.

Today, many healthcare organizations use national publications such as *Futurescan: Healthcare Trends and Implications 2011-2016* (Society for Healthcare Strategy and Market Development of the American Hospital Association 2011), which are updated annually, to kick off their review of changes in the external environment. Brief reviews of key local, regional, and state healthcare developments over the past year may also be prepared by the staff. Structured discussion about external and internal developments with senior management and/or the strategic planning committee is another important step in the environmental assessment update.

In an approach parallel to the full environmental assessment, the update typically produces three main outputs:

1. A revised set of competitive advantages and disadvantages
2. A revised set of assumptions about the future
3. A revised list of critical planning issues

ORGANIZATIONAL DIRECTION

Ordinarily, this component of the strategic plan requires the least attention in the annual update. Absent significant new developments (e.g., a merger, major acquisition, major divestiture or closure), the organizational direction components should remain largely intact from update to update. The mission and values statements are the most timeless and least likely to require modification. Even in today's tumultuous environment, the vision and principal strategy should last five to ten-plus years in most situations.

STRATEGY FORMULATION

There are two potential paths that may be followed here. If no change has occurred in the critical issues to be addressed, the focus of strategy formulation is exclusively on examining progress related to the plan's goals and objectives. Revisions may be warranted due to actual implementation success or failure, including pace of progress, roadblocks encountered, and the like. Revisions may also be warranted due to changes in environmental conditions.

A somewhat different approach is called for if new issues have been identified. In this case, strategy formulation also needs to include some processing of the new issue(s). This activity may be conducted in a manner similar to that followed in the complete planning process or, depending on current circumstances, in a less or more process-intensive fashion.

Much as in the environmental assessment, at a minimum senior management discusses and reviews strategy. Typically, the strategic planning committee is briefed and reviews the strategy outcomes.

IMPLEMENTATION PLANNING

This step proceeds in a manner similar to strategy formulation. If no new critical issues have been identified, the past year's action plans are reviewed and extended for another year, accounting for actual progress made, changed conditions, etc. Any new critical issue(s) and new goals and objectives developed for it will require development of an action plan for the next year with appropriate specificity (similar to the other action plans already in existence) and through appropriate processes.

At the conclusion of the annual update, board ratification of the new strategic plan is usually required. The scope and extent of the changes to the plan will ordinarily dictate how involved the approval process needs to be.

PROCESS OPTIONS FOR THE ANNUAL UPDATE

In nearly all cases, the process used in the annual update will be far less extensive than that employed in the initial development of the strategic plan or in the complete update that occurs when the plan has been accomplished.

Experience and observation suggest that the less turbulent the environment and the more the complete plan is on target and serving as a good road map for the organization, the less extensive the annual update process needs to be. When significant environmental change and concerns about the continuing relevance of key elements of the strategic plan emerge, a more extensive update process is required.

While there are seemingly infinite options for what to include in and how to carry out the annual update process, the options can be categorized into three general alternatives that represent points on the continuum of alternatives available.

1. **Least process.** Even in a relatively low-intensity update, some attention needs to be paid to each of the four strategic planning activities. At the minimalist end of the continuum, senior management and staff take responsibility for the majority of update activities, with modest input or participation from others. In this option, some outside input is generally sought in the external component of the environmental assessment to assist in validating the nature of current and expected future external conditions. Some internal input may also be sought in strategy formulation to fine-tune approaches to certain key issues. Planning committee involvement in the strategic planning process is also typically modest, limited to a few interactions with staff as they bring forward aspects of the updated plan.

2. **Moderate process.** In this option, more senior management and staff effort is required to complete the update and more input and participation is needed. This type of process usually results from one or more looming environmental threats (which have not occurred yet) or emerging concerns about the continued appropriateness of one or a few key strategies. A harder, more thorough review of the environment typically will be called for, or focused review and analysis of one or a few of the strategy elements in question may occur. More input and participation from those inside the organization, and potentially outside, is necessary. The planning committee's involvement in the update process is also greater.

3. **Most process.** With this option, something short of a full update is needed to address one or more major environmental changes that often are accompanied by additional threats of further change. Such change will typically call into question

key elements of the strategy; it is possible that elements of the strategy have already failed. In these situations, the update process will involve a fairly hard look at the environment, strategy, and implementation plans, and also may require a review of the organizational direction. Input and participation here is fairly extensive, often involving one or more task forces in strategy formulation and implementation planning as well as oversight by the planning committee throughout the update process.

Many organizations have found that planning retreats (see Chapter 7) are an excellent vehicle to accomplish a significant portion of the input and participation called for in the annual strategic plan update. Obviously, the need for and desirability of planning retreats vary somewhat depending on the scope and extent of the update required. Nevertheless, a growing number of healthcare organizations plan at least one annual strategic planning retreat as an important element of the annual update process.

LINKING THE ANNUAL UPDATE TO OTHER MANAGEMENT PROCESSES

As noted in Chapter 9 (see Exhibit 9.8), the annual strategic plan update should be integrated with financial and operational planning, ongoing strategic plan implementation, and opportunity testing. For most healthcare organizations the annual update occurs during the first half of the fiscal year. When beginning an annual update process, many healthcare organizations delay the start (and completion) of the process until later in the year and find that the necessary inputs for the budgeting process are not available in a timely manner. Experience indicates that an early start in the fiscal year for strategic plan updating provides for smoother integration with financial planning.

As a practical matter, the workflow needs to be staged and sequenced throughout the year so all elements of the management plans receive appropriate and thorough attention. Typically, the bulk of the work on the strategic plan update should be completed before financial and operating planning begins. But some flexibility must be built into the process so revisions of all plans can be made as necessary before finalization, depending on the results of each element of this process. During the third and (principally) fourth quarters, iterative revisions to the strategic, financial, and operating plans typically take place.

The annual update needs to interrelate with implementation of the previous year's strategic plan and ideas and opportunities that arise regularly between updates. As implementation occurs throughout the year, variation from what was envisioned will be called for and operationalized. New ideas and opportunities should be tested for their consistency with and relevance to the strategic plan. Some of these ideas and opportunities may be so compelling or emergent that they are implemented before the next plan update occurs. Others may be held for consideration at the time of the update. In any event, this routine management process could affect the annual update.

A FEW EXAMPLES

High Point Regional Health System

High Point Regional Health System (HPRHS) in High Point, North Carolina, has been using the annual update process for a number of years and illustrates well the many considerations that must be thought through in the update process. HPRHS consists of a 384-bed community and tertiary hospital, a number of ambulatory facilities, and other health services. Its annual budget is about $300 million (FY2009). HPRHS operates in the Greensboro-Winston Salem-High Point metropolitan market and competes primarily against three larger and quite successful systems: Novant Health, Wake Forest University Baptist Medical Center, and Moses Cone Health System.

HPRHS has employed the annual strategic planning process to stave off regular competitive thrusts by these well-heeled systems and identify opportunities that play off their weaknesses and HPRHS's strengths. Judging by its success over the past 15 years, HPRHS has done well, a fact that management attributes, at least in part, to its ongoing strategic planning efforts.

HPRHS's annual strategic plan update consists of three main process elements. First, senior management has an extended meeting shortly after the beginning of the fiscal year (October 1) to review and evaluate progress on the previous year's plan, analyze current and expected environmental conditions, and begin to formulate issues to be addressed in the annual update.

Second, a half-day mini-retreat is held with members of the strategic planning and finance committees of the board, typically in early December. This meeting results in confirmation of the issues to be dealt with in this planning cycle. The third major process element occurs about three months later and consists of a two-day retreat of the board, medical leadership, and management of HPRHS. In the time between the retreats, HPRHS's planning staff and senior management team formulate organizational direction and strategy. During the second retreat, a draft of the plan is presented to assembled leadership and, through a combination of large- and small- group review, the draft plan is reviewed and refined. After the retreat, planning staff and senior management complete the plan and receive formal board approval.

Commonwealth Medicine

A somewhat different approach is followed by Commonwealth Medicine (CWM). CWM is a $300+ million (annual revenue) division of the University of Massachusetts Medical School in

Worcester, Massachusetts. CWM's mission is "To distinguish the University of Massachusetts Medical School as a national leader in transforming publicly funded health care." To do this, CWM provides contract services, consulting, and research to public agencies and select other organizations to assist them in more effective performance of their roles.

CWM completed its last full strategic plan in 2006, and in 2011 is conducting a full review and revision. Since 2006 it has carried out a formal update each year. The update process starts when leadership convenes early in the year to formally assess progress in each of the six goal areas and to consider major changes in the environment (e.g., institution of universal health insurance in Massachusetts). Depending on the nature and extent of the challenges identified, either

- leadership charges a small steering committee with planning an annual retreat to be held two to three months later, or
- leadership convenes one or more work groups to address challenges that have been identified for discussion at a more extensive retreat under the aegis of the steering committee.

The retreat involves a broad group of CWM management staff, key collaborators from departments in the medical school, and other medical school leaders as appropriate. The retreat is an all-day session at a nearby, but off-site, location. At the retreat overall progress against plan is reviewed. Typically, the two to three areas that represent new challenges or where progress has been more difficult to achieve are discussed in a structured manner; recommendations for a new or revised course of action result from the retreat.

Following the retreat revisions are made to goals, new or revised objectives are developed, and action plans for all goals and objectives for the next year are established. Communication about the plan's changes and priorities are made to all managers, and through them, to all staff, in both written and oral form.

The structure, discipline, and regularity of the annual update process has allowed CWM to make good progress toward its stretch goals and vision over the past five years, where progress previously had been more difficult to realize and variable.

AtlantiCare

AtlantiCare is a medium-sized (about $700 million annual revenue) integrated delivery system in southeastern New Jersey. A Baldrige award winner in 2009, AtlantiCare has a lengthy history of effective strategic planning, but has modified its process in the past few years. With the completion of its 2008 long-term strategic plan, AtlantiCare moved to a rolling three-year strategic plan from the previously static five-year plan. This rolling process is integrated with its annual strategic planning process (see Exhibit 10.1). AtlantiCare believes that this approach "helps focus all levels of leadership on both the future direction of health care and the organization, while fostering flexibility, innovation, and agility in responding to a rapidly changing environment" (AtlantiCare 2011).

The move to a continuous, rolling strategic planning process is something that many other healthcare organizations are implementing or considering. As the environment becomes more dynamic, as noted in Chapter 9, a strategic management orientation is needed to address the interaction of the strategic, operational, and financial challenges healthcare organizations continuously face. AtlantiCare's strategic planning process evolution is a good illustration of how an organization can transition to this more sophisticated form of strategy management.

Exhibit 10.1: AtlantiCare Annual Strategic Planning Process (ASPP)

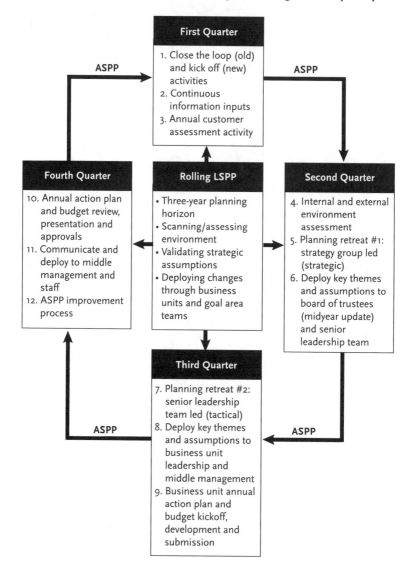

Note: LSPP = long-term strategic planning process

Source: AtlantiCare Malcolm Baldrige National Quality Award Application (2009). Used with permission.

CONCLUSION

How frequently are complete strategic planning efforts required versus the less intensive annual updates? The answer depends on the organization, its environment, its particular circumstances, and its style and culture. Over the past decade most healthcare organizations have prepared a comprehensive strategic plan about every three to five years, with the annual updates serving as the bridge between these larger efforts.

Most organizations recognize when the annual update is no longer sufficient to carry them forward effectively because the environment has changed markedly, the planning process has become stale, the organization has largely completed (or is substantially under way with) the major initiatives recommended in the last complete plan, or some combination of all three. Fogg (1994) indicates that a comprehensive update is required about every four to five years in the general business world, and healthcare organizations seem to be right in step with this timing.

CHAPTER 11

Encouraging Strategic Thinking

Beware of the 'Flavor of the Month.'

—*Linus Pauling*

Pursuing incremental improvement while rivals reinvent the industry is like fiddling while Rome burns.

—*Gary Hamel*

The hallmark of great companies is an ability to recognize the game has changed and to adapt.

—*Arthur Martinez quoted in* Brown and Eisenhardt

What your fiercest rival does badly, do incredibly well.

—*Umair Haque*

WHAT IS STRATEGIC THINKING?

This question is puzzling to most, if not all, healthcare executives and even strategic planning professionals. Only in the past decade has this question been addressed successfully outside healthcare.

Henry Mintzberg (1994), in his landmark devastating critique of strategic planning, said, "Strategic planning isn't strategic thinking. One is analysis, and the other is synthesis…[strategic thinking] involves intuition and creativity. The outcome of strategic thinking is an integrated perspective of the enterprise, a not-too-precisely articulated vision of direction…"

Garratt (1995) suggests that

Strategic thinking is essentially a process…to see, hear and use ingeniously the…signals which can give competitive advantage…It

Exhibit 11.1: Purposes of Strategic Thinking

In direction setting	"Locating, attracting, and holding customers is the purpose of strategic thinking" (Hickman and Silva 1984).
In establishing "the change agenda"	"Most organizations are effective in many of the things they do and deliver. Strategic thinking is about identifying what to change, modify, add, delete or acquire" (Kaufman 1991).
In resource allocation	"Strategic thinking is about making the best use of what will always be a limited amount and quality of resources" (Hanford 1983).

Source: Garratt, (1995). *Developing Strategic Thought*. Reproduced with permission of The McGraw-Hill Companies.

requires the ability to create a "holistic" view of the interconnections between apparently contradictory trends in [the] environment... and reframe the current mindsets which you and your competitors hold...."Strategic thinking" is the process by which an organization's direction-givers can rise above the daily managerial processes and crises to gain different perspectives of the internal and external dynamics causing change in their environment and thereby giving more effective direction to their organization.

Porter (1987) notes that "Strategic thinking rarely occurs spontaneously. Without formal planning systems, day-to-day concerns prevail. The future is forgotten. Formal planning provides the discipline to pause occasionally to think about strategic issues."

Hanford (1995) adds that "'Strategic thinking' in essence amounts to a richer and more creative way of thinking about and managing key issues and opportunities facing your organization....Strategic thinking underscores both the formulation and implementation of your organization's effective strategy" (see Exhibit 11.1).

Exhibit 11.2: Distinguishing Between Strategic and Operational Thinking

Strategic Thinking	Operational Thinking
• Longer term	• Immediate term
• Conceptual	• Concrete
• Reflective or learning	• Action or doing
• Identification of key issues and opportunities	• Resolution of existing performance problems
• Breaking new ground	• Routine and ongoing
• Effectiveness	• Efficiency
• "Hands off" approach	• "Hands on" approach
• "Helicopter" perspective	• "On the ground" perspective

Source: Hanford (1995) in Garratt (1995). *Developing Strategic Thought*. Reproduced with permission of The McGraw-Hill Companies.

While executives and board members may have a thorough understanding of and strong skills in operational thinking, Hanford (1995) argues that the needs are great for strong strategic thinking skills (see Exhibit 11.2), and far less has been done to develop these skills.

According to Swayne, Duncan, and Ginter (2008), "Strategic thinkers are always questioning: 'What are we doing now that we should stop doing?' 'What are we not doing now, but should start doing?' 'What are we doing now that we should continue to do but perhaps in a fundamentally different way?'" The Center for Applied Research (2001) suggests that "strategic thinking focuses on finding and developing unique opportunities to create value by enabling a provocative and creative dialogue among people who can affect a company's direction."

Mintzberg (1994) concludes that if strategic planning is to become truly effective and provoke serious organizational change, it needs to move beyond "preservation and rearrangement of established categories...and invent new ones....Formal planning has promoted strategies that are extrapolated from the past or copied from others....Strategy making needs to function beyond the boxes, to encourage the informal learning that produces new perspectives and new combinations."

How does an organization break out of the box and insert creativity, intuition, a future orientation, new perspectives, and new categories into its processes for and results from strategic planning? How can strategic planning better rise to Mintzberg's challenge and be a catalyst for critical organizational change?

STRATEGIC THINKING VERSUS STRATEGIC PLANNING

Robert (1998) suggests that "The strategic thinking process…can be described as the type of thinking that attempts to determine *what* an organization should look like in the future." Strategic planning, historically, has been primarily concerned with *how* to get there; operations is all about "how." Robert comments further: "Strategic thinking…identifies the key factors that dictate the direction of an organization, and it is a *process* that the organization's management uses to set direction and articulate their vision."

Robert (1998) believes there are four types of companies, as represented by the matrix in Exhibit 11.3.

1. Companies in the upper left quadrant exhibit strong strategic thinking and manage their operations well. Robert (1998) cites Walmart, Sony, and Johnson & Johnson as examples in this group.
2. Companies in the upper right quadrant have been successful through good operational management, but they cannot articulate where they are going. Robert believes that most US companies are in this group, as are 70 to 80 percent of all companies worldwide.
3. Companies in the lower left quadrant are excellent strategic thinkers, but they cannot implement their visions and generally are weak operationally. Robert believes that many personal computer manufacturers have historically fit into

Exhibit 11.3: The Strategic Thinking Matrix

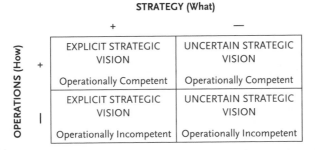

STRATEGY (What)

		+	−
OPERATIONS (How)	+	EXPLICIT STRATEGIC VISION Operationally Competent	UNCERTAIN STRATEGIC VISION Operationally Competent
	−	EXPLICIT STRATEGIC VISION Operationally Incompetent	UNCERTAIN STRATEGIC VISION Operationally Incompetent

Source: Robert (1998). *Strategy Pure and Simple II*. Reproduced with permission of The McGraw-Hill Companies.

this category and are now, as a result, defunct or merged into other companies.

4. Companies in the lower right quadrant exhibit the worst of both dimensions and usually do not survive very long. Robert (1998) cites Kmart as one example.

Robert (1998) suggests that strategic thinking skills are under-developed because most managers and board members have risen to the top ranks based on their skills in operations. In the course of their career development these individuals did not naturally develop the strategic skills necessary to help lead their companies, nor was much training or support in those areas provided to them.

THINKING DIFFERENTLY

Hamel and Prahalad (1995) state that,

To have a share in the future, a company must learn to think differently about three things: 1. the meaning of competitiveness, 2. the measuring of strategy, and 3. the meaning of organization....In many companies, strategic planning is essentially incremental tactical planning punctuated by heroic, and usually ill-conceived, investments….To avoid this situation, we need a concept of strategy that goes beyond form filling and blank cheque writing.

Hamel and Prahalad (1995) argue that strategic planning, as practiced in nearly all organizations, leads to incremental change at best, small gains in market share, and pursuit of modestly profitable niches. Strategic planning is far too focused on *what is*, rather than *what could be*. Deep debates or serious consideration of radical expansion of the boundaries of existing businesses rarely occur, and strategic planning fails to stretch far enough or question fundamental assumptions of the company and its senior staff. Given the rapid rate of change in most industries, strategic planning as described above is of marginal benefit. Hamel and Prahalad (1995) call for a more exploratory and less ritualistic planning process.

Hamel (1998) suggests five ways in which more insightful strategy might be brought forth.

1. Involve new voices in the conversation about strategy, including younger employees, new employees, and others outside the inner circle of senior leadership.
2. Create new conversations about strategy, involving diverse perspectives that cut across the usual organizational boundaries.
3. Ignite new passions among individuals involved in the change process that relate to their desires to grow professionally, share in the rewards of success, and have an instrumental role in creating a unique and exciting future.
4. Develop new perspectives about the company, its businesses, its competitors, and its customers that encourage new opportunities to emerge.
5. Encourage new experiments, particularly small-scale forays into new markets and businesses, to gain insights and learning about what strategies might work and which will not.

Above all, Hamel (1998) believes that senior staff must spend less time working on developing the perfect strategy and more time creating the conditions that could lead to strategy innovation: "In a discontinuous world, strategy innovation is the key to wealth creation. Strategy innovation is the capacity to reconceive the existing industry model in ways that create new value for customers, wrong-foot competitors, and produce new wealth for shareholders." The companies that have grown most successfully in the past decade or so have either invented new industries or dramatically reinvented existing ones. Their strategy is nonlinear.

Hamel (1996) characterizes linear strategy as ritualistic, reductionist, extrapolative, positioning, elitist, and easy. In exceptional (and unusual) companies the strategy is inquisitive, expansive, prescient, inventive, inclusive, and demanding. Hamel suggests that strategy making must become subversive and lead to revolution, not evolution, if it is to be an effective mechanism for leading change.

Eric Beinhocker and Sarah Kaplan (2002) provide a similar attack on conventional strategic planning and a call for new ways to reinvigorate strategic planning through improved strategic thinking processes. In an article whose title, "Tired of Strategic Planning," resonates with many senior executives, they note that "Many CEOs complain that their strategic-planning process yields few new ideas and is often fraught with politics" (Beinhocker and Kaplan 2002). They suggest that, consistent with Hamel's (1996) observations, a new process to make strategy is required. This process should have two primary goals.

1. **To build prepared minds**. If senior leaders gain a strong understanding of the business, the current and possible future environment, and the rationale for the organizational direction agreed on through the strategic planning process, they are more likely to be able to respond swiftly and effectively to challenges and opportunities that emerge.

2. **To build creative minds.** Beinhocker and Kaplan (2002) agree with Hamel (1996) that strategic experimentation is appropriate and will allow controlled testing about where future opportunities may be found. They also agree that many of the issues that companies face today are best addressed in multidisciplinary, cross-cutting forums that demand new voices, discussions, and perspectives.

NEW APPROACHES TO PROMOTE STRATEGIC THINKING

Businesses outside healthcare are years ahead of the healthcare industry in adopting approaches to promote strategic thinking in their organizations. Many companies have been using

- **contingency planning** to address a single uncertainty in a given situation;
- **sensitivity analysis** to examine the effect of a change in one variable while all other variables remain constant; and
- **simulation** to analyze the effects of simultaneous change in multiple variables.

SCENARIO PLANNING

An even more robust approach now employed increasingly frequently in healthcare is scenario planning. In contrast to contingency planning and sensitivity analysis, scenario planning allows for multiple changes in variables, incorporating both the objective analysis, which characterizes simulation, and subjective considerations more commonly found in the narrower approaches of contingency planning and sensitivity analysis.

According to Schoemaker (1995), "Scenario planning attempts to capture the richness and range of possibilities, stimulating decision makers to consider changes they would otherwise ignore. At the same time, it organizes those possibilities into narratives that are easier to grasp and use than great volumes of data."

Schoemaker (1995) indicates that scenario planning is particularly beneficial for organizations facing the following conditions:

- Uncertainty is high relative to managers' ability to predict or adjust.
- Many costly surprises have occurred in the past.
- The company does not perceive or generate new opportunities.
- The quality of strategic thinking is low (i.e., too routine or bureaucratic).
- The industry has experienced significant change or is about to.
- The company wants a common language and framework, without stifling diversity.
- There are strong differences of opinion, with multiple opinions having merit.
- The company's competitors are using scenario planning.

Schoemaker (1995) suggests that because scenarios are designed to construct possible futures but not specific strategies for dealing with them, some organizations find it beneficial to involve outsiders, such as major customers, key suppliers, regulators, consultants, and academics, in the scenario development process. The objective is "to build a shared framework for strategic thinking that encourages diversity and sharper perceptions about external changes and opportunities."

Schoemaker (1995) suggests a ten-step approach to scenario development:

1. Define the scope of scenarios to be developed, including time horizon and range. Look at past sources of uncertainty and volatility as guides.
2. Identify the major stakeholders who could influence the range of considerations defined in step 1.

3. Describe key future trends likely to affect the issues identified in step 1.
4. Identify major uncertainties that could significantly affect each issue.
5. Construct initial scenario themes.
6. Check for consistency and plausibility and revise scenario outlines as necessary.
7. Develop learning scenarios or the first full-scale version of the scenarios.
8. Identify research needs to flesh out uncertainties, trends, and blind spots in the learning scenarios.
9. Develop quantitative models, as appropriate, to better examine the interactions of certain variables.
10. Evolve toward discussion scenarios, through an iterative process, to converge on the final scenarios that will be used to test strategies and develop new ideas.

Schoemaker (1995) believes that good scenarios meet four tests: they are relevant, are internally consistent, describe clearly different futures, and are long term in perspective.

DECISION ANALYSIS AND GAME THEORY

Jennings, Clay, and Carr (2000) advocate the use of decision analysis and game theory as two additional techniques that have been used in business for many years to address future uncertainties creatively. While scenario planning is an excellent approach to address a large number of uncertainties, *decision analysis* works well when a limited number of possible alternatives exist. *Game theory* allows understanding of interdependencies among affected parties as a result of strategic initiatives, especially the reactions of competitors, strategic alliance partners, customers, and suppliers. These approaches are appropriate in many situations routinely encountered in strategic analysis and should become basic tools in the near future.

Exhibit 11.4: Value Innovation: The Cornerstone of Blue Ocean Strategy

Value innovation is created in the region where a company's actions favorably affect both its cost structure and its value proposition to buyers. Cost savings are made by eliminating and reducing the factors an industry competes on. Buyer value is lifted by raising and creating elements the industry has never offered. Over time, costs are reduced further as scale economies kick in due to the high sales volumes that superior value generates.

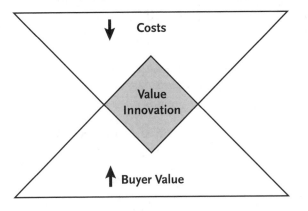

Source: Chan and Mauborgne (2005). Used with permission.

BLUE OCEAN STRATEGY

Kim and Mauborgne's (2005) research led to the coining of the term *blue ocean strategy* to describe the creation of uncontested market space. They argue that most companies pursue incremental improvements by attempting to outcompete their competitors and, in a zero sum game, increase their share of a crowded market. The more successful approach is to expand the boundaries of their market or invent entirely new market space, hence the term *blue ocean*.

These innovators do not use the competition as a reference point, but instead follow a different strategic logic they term *value innovation*. Value innovation, which defies the conventional competitive paradigm of having to choose between differentiation and cost, combines these two options to find new and uncontested market space (see Exhibits 11.4 and 11.5). This new space creates

Exhibit 11.5: Red Ocean Versus Blue Ocean Strategy

Red Ocean Strategy	Blue Ocean Strategy
Compete in existing market space.	Create uncontested market space.
Beat the competition.	Make the competition irrelevant.
Exploit existing demand.	Create and capture new demand.
Make the value-cost trade-off.	Break the value-cost trade-off.
Align the whole system of a firm's activities with its strategic choice of differentiation or low cost.	Align the whole system of a firm's activities in pursuit of differentiation and low cost.

Source: Chan and Mauborgne (2005). Used with permission.

opportunities for rapid and profitable growth versus the struggles in the traditional "red ocean" in which nearly all companies operate and compete. Kim and Mauborgne cite many examples of companies applying this kind of strategic thinking to the problem of crowded markets—Cirque du Soleil in the circus business is one recent example that clearly exemplifies this approach.

Kim and Mauborgne advise that blue ocean strategy contrasts with traditional strategic planning in the following ways:

- It should draw on collective wisdom, versus top-down or bottom-up planning.
- It focuses on building the big picture more than on number crunching.
- It should be conversational rather than documentation driven.
- It must be creative versus largely analytical.
- It should be motivational, resulting in "willing commitment," instead of bargaining driven, resulting in "negotiated commitment."

The bottom line, in their view, is to focus on how to break away from the competition, create blue ocean space, and then layer in the details of how to implement the strategy.

ADVANCED STRATEGIC THINKING

Academic and business journals present a growing body of literature on what could be characterized as advanced strategic thinking for those professionals who have a desire to learn more about this topic. Representative of this body of knowledge is the work of Hanford (1995). Hanford developed a program called Tools for Thinking Strategically (TTS), which is a skills-building and training program on this topic for trustees and executives. Hanford's program is designed to

- redefine or confirm the director's and executive's high-level role of setting direction by looking "outward, upward, and forward" to implement major changes and improvements;
- establish skills to formulate and successfully implement effective policies and strategies;
- develop a comfort level with assuming radically different behaviors;
- develop agility and adeptness in moving between strategic and operational behaviors by knowing when to be "in your helicopter" (acting strategically) versus being "on the ground" (acting operationally);
- assist individuals in becoming more personally effective in a variety of strategic support skill areas;
- build confidence about the ability to think strategically; and
- achieve constancy in strategic thinking as a result of more competence and confidence.

Hanford (1995) identifies four basic strategic thinking tools available to trustees and executives to enable them to think better in order to direct and manage better (see Exhibit 11.6).

1. **Thinking skills,** in which Hanford (1995) identifies four subtools:
   - Reframing, or developing one or more optional approaches to address an issue or opportunity (often by

Exhibit 11.6: Tools for Thinking Strategically

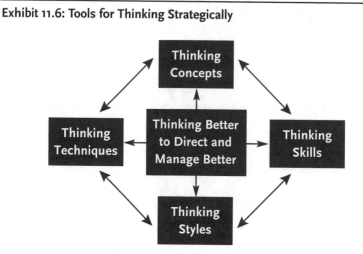

Source: Hanford (1995) in Garratt (1995). *Developing Strategic Thought.* Reproduced with permission of The McGraw-Hill Companies.

shifting the focus) rather than falling victim to "there's only one way to go."

- Map making, a deliberate approach to develop a full range of alternatives to address an issue before deciding what to do about it; this activity is accompanied by a collaborative approach—which includes developing the map and then deciding what to do about it—rather than the typical adversarial senior group discussion and decision-making process.
- Using searching questions to stimulate discussion of the "what ifs" and "why nots" in confronting the big issues facing the organization.
- Asking effective questions when reviewing issues to enhance creativity, increase commitment to organizational goals, and empower others to maximize their contributions to organizational success and their own job satisfaction.

2. **Thinking concepts**, in which Hanford identifies three sub-tools:
   - Holistic thinking to expand the breadth of individual and group thinking, based on the premise that the more fully you think about a situation, the better you can manage it.
   - Deeper thinking through the realization that results are dependent not only on effective actions but also on values, beliefs, and assumptions.
   - An expanded range of content thinking. Most director and executive content thinking can be categorized as "either/or" thinking (it is either "X" or it is "Y"); expand the range of alternatives to include "more/less" and "both/and" thinking. Similarly, most director and executive process thinking is "stay put" thinking, which is fine for straightforward issues in stable situations; expand the range of alternatives to include "minor from/to" and "major from/to" thinking.
3. **Thinking techniques**, in which Hanford identifies four sub-tools:
   - "Both/and." This involves thinking or explicit recognition of potential inconsistencies or tradeoffs in decision making and then creation of a map of the dilemma that can generate some approaches to resolve it.
   - Mind mapping. This process identifies the essential elements in achieving a strategic challenge and the interrelationships among the elements, which facilitates planning to meet the challenge.
   - Effective prioritization to reduce the number of important issues to deal with, based on urgency, relevance, growth, and ease of implementation, and to focus organizational resources to these priorities.
   - Choices and consequences thinking (also known as "more/less" thinking). This involves purposefully identifying alternative courses of action and then determining the relative merit of each alternative.

4. **Thinking styles**, in which Hanford identifies three subtools:
   - Revealing thinking intentions (or how you go about thinking). There are basically three thinking intentions: realize some new idea, describe what is true, or judge what is right. Recognizing this form of tunnel thinking allows development of an enriched and more balanced style for better decision making.
   - Identifying the kind of member a leader is. There are five types—synthesist, idealist, pragmatist, analyst, or realist. This tool expands thinking behavior to enhance decision making.
   - Understanding learning styles to improve how leaders learn, and promoting continuous improvement based on continuous learning.

Those who desire to know more about these concepts would benefit greatly from reading the source material on which this synopsis is based and then experimenting with one or more of the subtools. Goldman (2007) has also written extensively about how strategic thinking capabilities develop and how executives might become better strategic thinkers; her work is a cornerstone reference in this area.

CONCLUSION

Material presented in this chapter represents new thinking and behaviors for healthcare organizations and should be considered for adoption, especially given the increasing rate and pace of change in the field. Hanford (1995) suggests that in today's and tomorrow's increasingly difficult environment, directors and executives would be well advised to take "time out to increase your strategic thinking competencies. *Time spent thinking and learning how to think better is time well spent!*"

CHAPTER 12

Future Challenges for Strategic Planning and Planners

Change is the law of life. And those who look only to the past or present are certain to miss the future.

—John F. Kennedy

CONTINUOUS, ITERATIVE STRATEGIC PLANNING

In addition to all its other deficiencies, traditional strategic planning has been disparaged for being too static and linear in its processes. Today's faster pace of change and more turbulent environments render conventional approaches obsolete, according to critics. Part of this criticism has been addressed in Chapter 9, which describes the need to move organizations toward continuous strategic planning or, preferably, a strategic management process in contrast to periodic strategic planning. Criticisms about the linear nature of strategic planning are addressed below.

Begun and Heatwole (1999) and Krentz and Young (2000) advocate nonlinear or iterative strategic planning approaches (see Exhibits 12.1 and 12.2). In contrast to the traditional approach,

Exhibit 12.1: Strategic Cycling Model

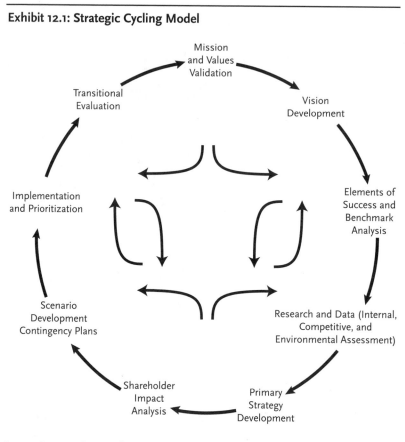

Source: Begun and Heatwole (1999). Used with permission.

where one step leads into the next and then the next and the next, with no backtracking, both authors suggest that the steps are so interrelated that strategic planning should proceed in a more iterative and, at times, nonlinear fashion.

Krentz and Young (2000) note that, "The steps in the process are likely to be intertwined. Although the organization ends up with outcomes that can be labeled 'the plan,' its thinking and deliberations are not linear, but more fluid in nature…"

Begun and Heatwole (1999) offer a different model, the "strategic cycling model." This "differs from other contemporary frame-

Exhibit 12.2: Linear Versus Fluid Planning Processes

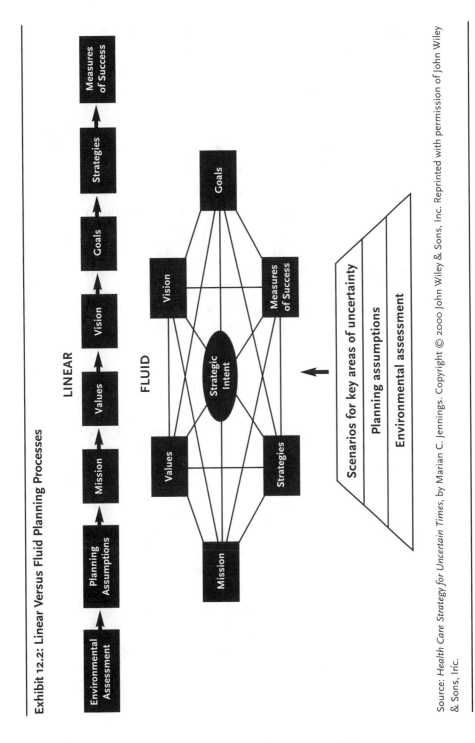

Source: *Health Care Strategy for Uncertain Times*, by Marian C. Jennings. Copyright © 2000 John Wiley & Sons, Inc. Reprinted with permission of John Wiley & Sons, Inc.

works in its emphasis on planning as a continuous feedback process rather than a set of stages that result in a relatively permanent and institutionalized plan....It represents a moving and flowing process of analysis and evaluation to continuously monitor the environment and adapt the organization."

As the environment grows more dynamic and unpredictable, strategic planning will need to evolve in the ways described by Begun and Heatwole (1999) and Krentz and Young (2000) to be more effective and useful. The approaches and processes described in this book move the traditional strategic planning methods a long way along the continuum toward the nonlinear and continuous end. In the evolution of their strategic planning approaches, healthcare organizations will need to be both iterative within a given cycle (per Begun and Heatwole and Krentz and Young) and merge planning into day-to-day operations so that regular and ongoing strategic management occurs, as discussed in Chapter 9.

THE NEW STRATEGIC PLANNER

These new perspectives about healthcare strategic planning argue for careful reconsideration of the role of the strategic planner in guiding and shaping the strategic planning process. Hiam (1993) (see Exhibit 12.3) notes that

> A recent survey by Business International found that planners currently perform ten principal functions, which range from gathering information for top managers to serving as "guardians" of the planning process. These can be divided into three basic categories: information functions, facilitation functions, and process management functions....Unfortunately, this list of current planning functions doesn't dovetail too well with the strategy needs of organizations in highly turbulent environments.

Exhibit 12.3: The Old Guard Versus the New Breed

The Old Guard	The New Breed
Strategic planners' traditional functions, according to a Business International survey, were well defined:	*It can be a struggle for organizations to keep up with an increasingly complex business world. The role of strategic planners should therefore evolve within the framework of traditional functions and be updated with new functions designed to teach organizations to transform themselves:*
Information functions:	**Information functions:**
• Compile information for top managers.	• Compile information for all strategy-oriented teams.
• Research competitors.	• Research competitors and best-in-class benchmarks, including noncompetitors.
• Prepare forecasts.	• Prepare forecasts, especially on internal changes in culture and management style and their effects on environment and performance.
Facilitation functions:	**Facilitation functions:**
• Consult with divisions on how to prepare plans and strategies.	• Consult with divisions on how to improve performance through education, innovation, process management, and total quality management.
• Standardize reporting formats and create common terms of reference.	• Help divisions measure cost of quality, management effectiveness, and team progress.
• Help senior managers convey corporate culture by working cultural factors into the planning process.	• Help senior managers implement changes in corporate culture and measure the impact on performance.
• Communicate corporate objectives.	**Process management functions:**
• Organize and lead planning teams.	• Manage the expansion of the planning process and encourage intelligent employee participation.
Process management functions:	• Develop a process-management methodology and oversee its application to all business processes.
• Manage the planning process.	**Transformation functions:**
• Develop new planning methods.	• Add an internal element (one that asks how to improve as well as what to focus on) to the traditional, externally focused strategic plan. The plan should identify needs and set goals in areas such as management development, benchmarking, process improvement, culture change, and employee participation.
	• Push for recognition that the annual planning cycle is too long, and forecasts too weak, to permit pursuit of a single strategy. Build mechanisms for reassessment into the strategic plan and the organization as a whole.
	• Develop new ways to measure organizational capabilities and performance, focusing on sources of strategic advantage, such as organizational learning rate.

Source: Hiam (1993). Used with permission.

Hiam (1993) believes that planners need to take on a new role that is "participative, missionary and aggressively iconoclastic… and [become] active participants and leaders in the transformation of management" and their organizations (see Exhibit 12.3).

Mintzberg (1994) argues similarly that the new role of strategic planners consists of three elements:

1. **Planners as strategy finders**. Planners need to be active searchers for key strategies that emerge within top management, often unintentionally or even without management awareness. Planners need to be constantly on the prowl to discover these "amid the ruin of failed experiments, seemingly random activities, and messy learning" (Mintzberg 1994). Planners should be alert to activities both inside and outside their organizations that can lead to new, important strategies.

2. **Planners as analysts**. Planners have traditionally performed this role of analysis and are quite comfortable with it. However, Mintzberg (1994) suggests that planners need to have a broader view of their role in analytical support to offer new models, conceptual approaches, and new processes to address problems.

3. **Planners as catalysts**. Similar to Hiam's (1993) recommendation that planners assume a management and organizational transformation role, Mintzberg (1994) believes that planners need to "encourage managers to think about the future in creative ways. Such planners see their job as getting others to question conventional wisdom and especially helping people out of conceptual ruts."

Finally, Beckham (2000) writes that the successful CEO of the future needs to be a "master strategist" or have such a person as a key staff member. Whether a strategic planner or the CEO assumes this role directly, Beckham (2000) believes the effective strategist exhibits five principal qualities:

1. **A high percentage of right calls**. While all senior managers need to pitch in when predicting the future, one or more may have a better track record and a clearer crystal ball than others and should be relied on as a primary resource.
2. **Innovativeness**. An ability to break away from current thinking and embrace a new view.
3. **Introspection and learning**. An ability to learn from experience, both successes and failures.
4. **Confidence, resolve, and patience**. An ability to let strategies play out, through various ups and downs as they emerge, to realize the potential benefits of change.
5. **Watchfulness and listening**. An ability to carefully watch and listen and not feel the need to dominate or steer every conversation or discussion.

The effective strategic planner and strategist of the future is much more than an information gatherer or guardian of the planning process. He or she is a leader in management and organizational transformation, a multidimensional catalyst of organizational change, and a strategy finder, enabler, and leader. This transformational agenda is ambitious for many healthcare strategic planners, but carries huge potential for personal and professional growth and success.

A study conducted by Health Strategies & Solutions, Inc., and the Society for Healthcare Strategy & Market Development in 2005 to 2006 (Zuckerman 2007) reports that planners and executives believe that healthcare strategic planning practices are effective and provide the appropriate focus and direction for their organizations. Fundamental strategic planning practices appear to be sound, with strategic planning being well accepted, used regularly, and integrated increasingly well with other management functions.

But when compared to strategic planning practices outside of the healthcare field, it is clear that healthcare strategic planning has not advanced to the more sophisticated levels seen outside of healthcare and is far behind what are considered state-of-the-art practices. In fact, the areas where healthcare organizations seem to do best according to the survey results—development of mission statements, participation of senior management in the planning process, and development of goals—are rudimentary in strategic planning outside of the healthcare field. Organizations exhibiting more advanced strategic planning would merely think of these areas as the basics, not best practices or even strengths.

Companies that demonstrate pathbreaking strategic planning practices outside of healthcare already embody what are considered best practice strategic planning approaches among healthcare providers today, such as attacking critical issues, developing clear strategies, achieving real benefits, and managing implementation.

More important, outside of healthcare, planning practices at pathbreaking companies are characterized by the following five qualities:

1. **Systematic, ongoing internal and external data gathering that leads to the use of knowledge management practices.**
   Rather than the ad hoc data assembly and analysis frequently observed in healthcare organizations, pathbreaking companies outside of healthcare have highly structured systems for continuously gathering information that drives strategic planning. Data gathered are of a breadth and depth rarely seen among healthcare organizations. Once data are gathered, nonlinear analysis is conducted using sophisticated modeling, game theory, and other advanced approaches that far exceed the linear techniques and correlations used in healthcare organizations. The most advanced companies take these efforts to even higher levels by using knowledge management programs that sort information into databases and allow easy access and use by personnel at all levels throughout the organization. Data collection and analysis focus on the market and external factors and forces so that decision making is largely driven from the outside versus inside, as is now common in healthcare organizations.

2. **Innovation and creativity are prized charact[...]
   strategic planning.** Pathbreaking companies [...]
   high value they place on innovation and creat[...]
   a work environment that is receptive to new [...]
   at alternatives, especially when they create ne[...]
   market space. Risk-averse healthcare providers unaci̇sca[...]
   the concepts of innovation and creativity, but putting them
   into action is another matter. The key issue here is less one of
   "what to do," but rather "how to do it." Demonstrating leadership instead of followership and becoming risk tolerant are
   important first steps for healthcare organizations. Developing
   a culture that supports, or better yet, encourages risk taking is
   a necessary prerequisite to progress.

3. **Strategic planning is more bottom up than top down.**
   Leading firms outside of healthcare use a planning process
   that is increasingly focused in the business units or subsidiaries, with corporate leadership providing high-level direction.
   This approach allows strategic planning to be more broad
   based, meaningful, and substantial, with the "real" action of
   planning taking place closer to the customer. More organizational support for initiatives is nurtured when planning has
   a bottom-up orientation, and implementation may be more
   successful when planning has been vigorous at lower levels of
   the organization. Healthcare strategic planning is still mostly
   a top-down process that engenders little participation, awareness, or support from the majority of employees.

4. **Evolving, flexible, and continuously improving strategic
   planning processes help organizations adapt more readily.**
   Pathbreaking companies embrace the inevitability of change
   and use planning processes with an external orientation. They
   use external forces and factors to create a platform for change
   that keeps planning responsive and vital. They regularly revise
   and upgrade their planning processes and techniques based
   on their own experiences, observations of other leading companies, and academic research in the field. Many healthcare

organizations are content to use the tried and true strategic planning processes that worked well historically. Most healthcare professionals are not content with yesterday's operations management and financial planning approaches, so why shouldn't they support similar levels of change in their strategic planning processes?

5. **Dynamic strategic planning has replaced static planning.** Many companies in rapidly changing industries recognize that strategic planning must be dynamic—vision statements must inspire and stretch the organization, goals may need to be revolutionary, strategic thinking is encouraged, decision making is driven down to all levels, and strategic planning is embedded throughout the culture. Strategic planning becomes everyone's job, every day, not just an annual or periodic exercise by executive leaders.

Healthcare leaders must look beyond their own backyards to learn how other highly competitive industries are moving their organizations to higher levels of growth and success with more rigorous and sophisticated planning. The five qualities discussed here, even when executed at rather basic levels, will go a long way toward helping healthcare organizations experience the benefits that path-breaking companies realize from their planning processes.

CONCLUSION

The good old days of the relatively calm and stable healthcare environment are long gone. Intuition and educated guesses are no longer viable substitutes for sound planning methods. Change is occurring so rapidly that it is impossible to fully understand its scope and impact. With organizations no longer able to rely on the accuracy of long-range forecasts, they must improve their ability to respond to unanticipated changes in the market.

The question is, How will change be experienced? According to Hamel and Prahalad (1994), organizations have two choices:

> Given that change is inevitable, the real issue for managers is whether that change will happen belatedly, in a crisis atmosphere, or with foresight, in a calm and considered manner; whether the transformation agenda will be set by a company's more prescient competitors or by its own point of view; whether the transformation will be spasmodic and brutal or continuous and peaceful.

To quote George Bernard Shaw, "To be in hell is to drift, to be in heaven is to steer." Strategic planning is the vehicle that enables healthcare organizations to steer and have control over their future. Yet strategic planning is a journey without a specific destination. It will take soul searching, courage, and commitment to face a future full of uncertainty and potential threats. Strategic planning can provide the road map to guide organizations through the unknown, balancing the need for articulated and compelling vision and direction with the flexibility to adapt and respond as healthcare is transformed in the coming years.

References

Ascension Health. 2011. "Strategic Direction." Accessed 1/11/12.
www.ascensionhealth.org/index.php?option=com_content&vi
ew=article&id=14&Itemid=127.

AtlantiCare. 2011. Malcolm Baldrige National Quality Award
Application. Accessed 5/3/11. www.atlanticare.org/about/
baldrige.php

Barnes-Jewish Hospital. 2011. "Mission, Vision & Values."
Accessed 1/11/12. www.barnesjewish.org/about/
mission-vision-values.

Bart, C. K. 2002. "Creating Effective Mission Statements." *Health
Progress* (September/October): 41.

Beckham, J. D. 2000. "Strategy: What It Is, How It Works, Why
It Fails." *Health Forum Journal* 43 (6): 55–59.

Begun, J., and K. B. Heatwole. 1999. "Strategic Cycling: Shaking Complacency in Healthcare Strategic Planning." *Journal of Healthcare Management* 44 (5): 339–51.

Begun, J. W., and A. A. Kaissi. 2005. "An Exploratory Study of Healthcare Strategic Planning in Two Metropolitan Areas." *Journal of Healthcare Management* 50 (4): 264–75.

Beinhocker, E. D., and S. Kaplan. 2002. "Tired of Strategic Planning?" *McKinsey Quarterly* (2): 1–7.

Bellenfant, W. L., and M. J. Nelson. 2010. "Improving Performance Through Execution of Strategy." Financial Resource Group. Accessed 8/11/10. http://frgroup.net/articles/article_strategic_planning.pdf.

———. 2002. "Strategic Planning: Looking Beyond the Next Move." *Healthcare Financial Management* (October): 63.

Bossidy, L., and R. Charan. 2002. *Execution: The Discipline of Getting Things Done.* New York: Crown Publishing Group.

Bracker, J. 1980. "The Historical Development of the Strategic Management Concept." *Academy of Management Review* 5 (2): 219–24.

Brown, S. L., and K. M. Eisenhardt. 1998. *Competing on the Edge.* Boston: Harvard Business School Press.

Bruton, G. D., B. M. Oviatt, and L. Kallas-Bruton. 1995. "Strategic Planning in Hospitals: A Review and Proposal." *Healthcare Management Review* 20 (3): 16–25.

Campbell, A. B. 1993. "Strategic Planning in Health Care: Methods and Applications." *Quality Management in Health Care* 1 (4): 13.

Center for Applied Research. 2001. "Briefing Notes: What Is Strategic Thinking?" Accessed 1/4/11. www.cfar.com/Documents/strathink.pdf.

Chan, K. W., and R. Mauborgne. 2005. *Blue Ocean Strategy.* Boston: Harvard Business School Press.

Clark, T. R. 2011. "The Power of Vision Provides Organizations with Direction, Inspiration." *Deseret News* (February 14). www.deseretnews.com/article/705366518/The-power-of-vision-provides-organizations-with-direction-inspiration.html.

Coile, R. C., Jr. 1994. "Making Strategic Planning a Vision-Driven Process." *Hospital Strategy Report* 6 (10): 8.

Collins, J. 1995. "Building Companies to Last." Accessed 11/18/11. www.jimcollins.com/article_topics/articles/building-companies.html.

Collins, J., and J. Porras. 1996. "Building Your Company's Vision." *Harvard Business Review* (September). Accessed 11/18/11. www.tecker.com/downloads/buildingvision.pdf.

Community Health Systems. 2010. "Strategies to Success." Accessed 1/11/12. www.chs.net/company_overview/strategies.html.

Corboy, M., and D. O'Corribui. 1999. "The Seven Deadly Sins of Strategy." *Management Accounting* 77 (10): 29–30.

Drucker, P. F. 1999. *Management Challenges for the 21st Century.* New York: HarperBusiness.

———. 1998. "Four Challenges to Received Wisdom." Accessed 1/11/12. www.mastersforum.com/PastPrograms/PeterDruckerAConversationwithPeterDrucker/tabid/62/Default.aspx.

Dye, R., O. Sibony, and S. P. Viguerie. 2009. "Strategic Planning: Three Tips for 2009." *McKinsey Quarterly.* Accessed 3/16/11. www.mckinseyquarterly.com/Strategic_planning_Three_tips_for_2009_2340?pagenum=2.

Einblau, R. 2003. "Strategic Planning in Turbulent Times." *Canadian Business and Current Affairs* 59 (10): 6–8.

Evashwick, C. J., and W. T. Evashwick. 1988. "The Fine Art of Strategic Planning." *Provider* 14 (4): 4–6.

Fogg, C. D. 1994. *Team-Based Strategic Planning: A Complete Guide to Structuring, Facilitating, and Implementing the Process.* New York: American Management Association.

Garratt, R. (ed.). 1995. *Developing Strategic Thought: Rediscovering the Art of Direction-Giving.* London: McGraw-Hill.

Goldman, E. 2007. "Strategic Thinking at the Top." *MIT Sloan Management Review* 48 (4): 75–81.

Google. 2011. "Company." Accessed 9/19/11. www.google.com/about/corporate/company.

Griffith, J. R., and J. A. Alexander. 2002. "Measuring Comparative Hospital Performance." *Journal of Healthcare Management* 47 (1): 42–43.

Hamel, G. 1998. "Strategy Innovation and the Quest for Value." *Sloan Management Review* 39 (2): 7.

———. 1996. "Strategy as Revolution." *Harvard Business Review* 74 (4): 69–82.

Hamel, G., and C. K. Prahalad. 1995. "Thinking Differently." *Business Quarterly* 59 (4): 22–24.

———. 1994. "Competing for the Future." *Harvard Business Review* 72 (4): 122–28.

Hanford, P. 1995. "Developing Director and Executive Competencies in Strategic Thinking." In *Developing Strategic Thought: Rediscovering the Art of Direction-Giving*, edited by R. Garratt, 157–84. London: McGraw-Hill.

———. 1983. "Managing for Results." Unpublished paper written for the Public Service Board, Queensland State Government, Brisbane, Australia.

Haque, U. 2010. "Strategy's Golden Rule." HBR Blog Network. Accessed 5/12/11. http://blogs.hbr.org/haque/2010/04/strategys_golden_rule.html.

Hiam, A. 1993. "Strategic Planning Unbound." *Journal of Business Strategy* 14 (2): 46–52.

Hickman, C., and M. Silva. 1984. "On Becoming a Strategic Thinker." In *Creating Excellence: Managing Corporate Culture, Strategy and Change in the New Age.* London: George Allen and Unwin.

Hunterdon Healthcare System. 2011. "The Hunterdon Healthcare System." Accessed 9/19/11. www.hunterdonhealthcare.org/about.asp.

Inamdar, N. 2002. "Applying the Balanced Scorecard in Healthcare Provider Organizations." *Journal of Healthcare Management* 47 (3): 179.

Institute of Medicine (IOM). 1999. *To Err Is Human.*
Washington, DC: National Academies Press.

Jennings, M. C., S. B. Clay, and E. Carr. 2000. "Tools to Address
Uncertainty." In *Health Care Strategy for Uncertain Times*, edited
by M. Jennings; 99-134. Chicago: Jossey-Bass/AHA Press.

Joint Commission, The. 2009. "The Joint Commission Mission
Statement." Published August 15. www.jointcommission.org/
the_joint_commission_mission_statement.

Kaplan, R., and D. Norton. 1996. "Using the Balanced Scorecard
as a Strategic Management System." *Harvard Business Review*
74 (1): 75–85.

Kaplan, R. S., D. P. Norton, and E. A. Barrows. 2008. *Developing
the Strategy: Vision, Value Gaps, and Analysis.* Boston: Harvard
Business School Publishing.

Kaufman, R. 1991. *Strategic Planning Plus: An Organization
Guide.* Newbury Park, CA: Sage Publications.

Kim, W. C., and R. Mauborgne. 2005. *Blue Ocean Strategy: How
to Create Uncontested Market Space and Make Competition
Irrelevant.* Boston: Harvard Business Review Press.

Kouzes, J. M., and B. Z. Posner. 1996. "Envisioning Your Future:
Imagining Ideal Scenarios." *Futurist* 30(3): 14–19.

Krentz, S. E., and J. S. Young. 2000. "Strategy Formulation in
Health Care." In *Health Care Strategy for Uncertain Times*,
edited by M. Jennings, 19–38. Chicago: Jossey-Bass/AHA
Press.

Mankins, M. C., and R. Steele. 2005. "Turning Great Strategy Into
Great Performance." *Harvard Business Review* 83 (7/8) 64–72.

McKinsey Quarterly. 2006. *Improving Strategic Planning: A
McKinsey Survey.* Accessed 2/12/11. www.mckinseyquarterly
.com/Improving_strategic_planning_A_McKinsey_Survey_1819.

Memorial Health System. 2011. "About MHS." Accessed 1/11/12.
www.choosememorial.org/About/Default.aspx.

Miles, R. E., and C. C. Snow. 1978. *Organizational Strategy,
Structure, and Process.* New York: McGraw-Hill.

Mintzberg, H. 1994. "The Fall and Rise of Strategic Planning." *Harvard Business Review* 72 (1): 107–13.

Nadler, D. A. 1994. "Collaborative Strategic Thinking." *Planning Review* 22 (5): 30.

Nike, Inc. 2011. "What Is Nike's Mission Statement?" Accessed 9/19/11. http://help-us.nike.com/app/answers/detail/a_id/113.

Porter, M. E. 1996. "What Is Strategy?" *Harvard Business Review* (November–December): 61–78.

———. 1987. "The State of Strategic Thinking." *The Economist* (May 23): 18.

———. 1980. *Competitive Strategy.* New York: Free Press.

Rheault, D. 2003. "Freshening Up Strategic Planning: More Than Fill-in-the-Blanks." *Journal of Business Strategy* 24 (16): 33–35.

Robert, M. 1998. *Strategy Pure and Simple II: How Winning Companies Dominate Their Competitors,* revised edition. New York: McGraw-Hill.

Romero, J. L. 2011. "Vision Statement Examples." Accessed 1/18/11. www.skills2lead.com/vision-statement-examples.html.

Schoemaker, P. J. H. 1995. "Scenario Planning: A Tool for Strategic Thinking." *Sloan Management Review* 36 (2): 25–41.

Sentara Healthcare. 2011. "About Sentara Healthcare." Accessed 1/11/12. www.sentara.com/aboutsentara/Pages/AboutSentara.aspx?P.

Simyar, F., J. Lloyd-Jones, and J. Caro. 1988. "Strategic Management: A Proposed Framework for the Health Care Industry." In *Strategic Management in the Health Care Sector: Toward the Year 2000,* edited by F. Simyar and J. Lloyd-Jones, 6–17. Englewood Cliffs, NJ: Prentice Hall.

Society for Healthcare Strategy and Market Development of the American Hospital Association. 2011. *Futurescan Healthcare Trends and Implications 2011–2016.* Chicago: Health Administration Press.

Sorkin, D. L., N. B. Ferris, and J. Hudak. 1984. *Strategies for Cities and Counties: A Strategic Planning Guide.* Washington, DC: Public Technology, Inc.

Spiegel, A. D., and H. H. Hyman. 1991. *Strategic Health Planning Methods and Techniques Applied to Marketing and Management*. Norwood, NJ: Ablex Publishing Corp.

Swayne, L. E., W. J. Duncan, and P. M. Ginter. 2008. *Strategic Management of Health Care Organizations*, sixth edition. West Sussex, UK: John Wiley & Sons Ltd.

Taub, S. 2003. "Is Planning a Waste of Time?" Accessed 1/11/12. www.cfo.com/article.cfm/3010159?f=related.

Webster, J. L., W. R. Reif, and J. S. Bracker. 1989. "The Manager's Guide to Strategic Planning Tools and Techniques." *Planning Review* 17 (6): 5.

Wells, D. L. 1996. *Strategic Management for Senior Leaders: A Handbook for Implementation*. Publication # 96-03. Arlington, VA: Department of the Navy Total Quality Leadership Office.

Zuckerman, A. M. 2007. *Raising the Bar: Best Practices for Healthcare Strategic Planning*. Chicago: Society for Healthcare Strategy & Market Development.

———. 2005. "Executing Your Strategic Plan." *H&HN Online*. Accessed 1/11/12. www.hhnmag.com/hhnmag_app/jsp/articledisplay.jsp?dcrpath=HHNMAG/PubsNewsArticle/data/050607HHN_Online_Zuckerman&domain=HHNMAG.

Index

Ascension Health, St. Louis, Missouri, strategy statement of, 72

Atlanticare, strategic plan updating process of, 201–202

B

Balanced Scorecard Collaborative, 169

Balanced scorecards, 180–185; business planning component of, 184; communication and linking component of, 184; definition of, 180, 182; development of, 182, 183; feedback component of, 184, 185; implementation of, 182, 183; learning component of, 184, 185; as strategic management tools, 187; use in strategic plan implementation, 180–185; vision component of, 181, 182, 184

Balance sheets, management of, 156, 158, 159

Barnes-Jewish Hospital, St. Louis, Missouri: mission statement of, 63; vision statement of, 66

Barrett, Colleen C., 103

BC (British Columbia) Children's Hospital: key strategic planning issues for, 53; mission statement of, 72; organizational direction statement of, 72; strategy

statement of, 71, 72; vision statement of, 72

Benefits, of strategic planning, 1–2, 11–13, 151–167; community benefits, 152–153, 163–167; financial improvement, 152–153, 155–159, 167; identification of benefits, 152–155; operational improvement, 152–153, 159–163, 167; product and market improvement, 152–155, 167; understanding of, 173

Best practices, in strategic planning, 227–230

Blue ocean strategy, 215–216

Board, roles in strategic planning, 23, 24, 105, 142, 144; facilitation, 25; mission statement development, 62–63, 64; organizational direction, 61; strategic plan approval, 114, 117–118; strategic plan implementation, 173; strategic plan review, 113, 117–118; teamwork, 135

Bond ratings, 46

Bossidy, Larry, 169

Business International, 224

Buttonwood Group, 5

C

Capital, use of, 156, 157–158

Capital projects, 157–158; funding for, 157

Community leaders, role in strategic planning, 146

Companies. *See also specific companies:* pathbreaking, 228–230; strategic thinking skills of, 208–209

Competition: blue ocean strategy response to, 215–216; from for-profit niche providers, 7; impact on strategic planning, 6; increase in, 16–17; from physician entrepreneurs, 7; between physicians and hospitals, 142–143

Competitive advantages, 46–48

Competitive disadvantages, 46–48

Competitive strategy, 4

Competitor data, sources of, 42

Competitors, environmental analysis of, 42, 43, 44–45

Consensus, in strategic planning, 132, 138; failure of, 15

Consultants: in scenario planning, 213; in strategic planning, 133

Consulting practices, 157

Consumer-driven healthcare, 21

Content ("either/or") thinking, 219

Contingency planning/plans, 7, 89–90, 91, 119; for healthcare reform, 89, 91; as implementation framework component, 110; implemen-

tation of, 187; for promotion of strategic thinking, 212

Continuity of care, 154, 155

Coordination, 12, 21, 143

Corporations. *See also* Companies; *specific* corporations: strategic planning by, 3–5

Cost leadership strategy, 70

Creativity, receptivity to, 228–229

Critical planning issues: examples of, 81; failure to identify, 15; identification of, 51–55, 79–81; relationship to goals, 85, 86; white papers on, 81–83, 85

D

Dartmouth Atlas of Health Care, 36

Data: historical, 26–27, 37; online sources of, 36

Data analysis: excessive, 35; nonlinear, 228

Data collection: of competitor data, 42; with focus groups, 141; guidelines for, 35–37; with interviews, 140; with reactor panels, 141; with surveys, 140; systemic and ongoing, 228

Decision analysis, 214

Decision making, strategic planning as, 3

Defenders, 69, 70

Dell, Michael, 77

Demographic indicators, trends analysis of, 40–41, 43, 45

Designing and Conducting Survey Research: A Comprehensive Guide (Rea and Parker), 140

Development tasks. *See* Transitioning to implementation

Differentiation strategy, 70–71

Digital Equipment Corporation, 49

Direction, organizational. *See* Organizational direction

Disadvantages, competitive, 46–48

Discontinuation, of programs or services, 101, 102

Disney, values statement of, 74

Downsizing, of programs or services, 101, 102

Drucker, Peter, 62, 151

Dynamic healthcare environment, responsiveness to, 16

E

Economic indicators, trends analysis of, 40–41, 43, 45

Emergency departments, operational improvement of, 160, 161, 163

Endowments, 157

Environmental assessments, 7, 8, 9, 10, 33–56; components of, 8, 9, 10, 33–35; data requirements for, 36; external, 8, 9, 37, 40–55; final

tasks in, 51–55; future focus of, 48–51; goal of, 8; identification of critical issues in, 51–55; internal, 37–40, 46–55; organizational review in, 8, 9; poor planning and execution of, 35; purposes of, 35; updating of, 119, 193–194

Equipment, internal assessment of, 39

"Executing Your Strategic Plan" (Zuckerman), 173

Execution, of strategic plans. *See* Implementation, of strategic plans

Executive summaries, 111, 112–113; distribution of, 113–114; examples of, 113, 114–116; integration into strategic plans, 112; length of, 112; as stand-alone documents, 112; submission of, 88

Experimentation, strategic, 212

External assessment, 8, 9; approach to, 40–45; end product of, 45–46; key outputs of, 46–55

F

Facilitation, in strategic planning, 132–135; identification of facilitators for, 25; skills required for, 133–135; team interventions in, 136

Facilities, internal assessment of, 39

169–172; progress monitoring and review of, 104, 105, 119, 173, 175, 176–180; rewards for achievement of, 179–180; timing of, 110

Implementation subcommittees, 174–175

Implementation team members, 105–106, 110

Income, nonoperating, 156, 157

Income statements, projected baseline, 99

Information gathering. *See* Data collection

Initiatives: identification of, 78, 85–88; net financial impact of, 100; prioritization of, 86, 87, 88

Innovation, 211; receptivity to, 228–229; value, 215–216

Innovativeness, of strategic planners, 227

Institute of Medicine, *To Err Is Human* report of, 161

Integration strategy, 71

Internal assessments, 8, 9; approach to, 37–40; end product of, 40; key outputs of, 46–55; SWOT use in, 37–40

International Business Machines (IBM), 49

Internet, surveys conducted on, 140

Interviews, 140; as market research tool, 43

Introspection, 227

J

Johnson & Johnson, 208

Joint Commission, 60

Joint Commission Quality Check, 42

K

Kanter, Rosabeth Moss, 131

Kaplan, Robert, 180, 185

Kennedy, John F., 221

Kickoff retreats, 137

Knowledge management programs, 228

L

Lakein, Alan, 1

Leaders/leadership, in strategic planning, 22-23, 171. *See also* Facilitation, in strategic planning: absence of, 111; of annual strategic plan updating, 200; of implementation progress review meetings, 179; of strategic plan implementation, 110–111, 173, 174, 179; thinking styles of, 220

Learning: balanced scorecard assessment of, 181, 182; from experience, 227

Learning styles, 220

Leeds University, 59

LeGuin, Ursula, 131

Listening skills, of strategic planners, 227

M

Managed care, impact on strategic planning, 6

Management: lack of, 172; of strategic plan implementation, 172, 175–176, 185–188

Management action plans, 88

Management structures, internal assessment of, 38

Management tools, strategy *versus*, 59–60

Map making, 218

Market benefits, of strategic planning, 152–155, 167

Market forecasts, external assessment of, 43, 45

Market research: as external assessment task, 42–43; as internal assessment task, 43; primary, 39, 42–43; purposes of, 39, 42–43

Market segments, identification of, 4

Market (service) areas, 153, 154

Market share, 46, 48, 154, 155

Market space, new and uncontested, 215–216

Martinez, Arthur, 205

McKinsey Quarterly, 5

Medical executive committees, strategic plan review by, 117

Medical staff leadership, strategic plan review by, 117

Meetings: orientation, 29; for strategic plan progress review, 177, 179

Memorial Health System, Springfield, Illinois: action plan progress reviews by, 178; values statement of, 74

Merger strategies, 7

Microprocess retreats, 138

Middle management, as strategic plan implementation team, 105–106, 110

Milne, A.A., 19

Mimicry, avoidance of, 30

Mind mapping, 219

Mission, 3

Mission statements: characteristics of, 62; definition of, 62; development of, 61–64, 227–228; as directional strategy, 57–58; duration of, 194; examples of, 62, 63, 113; as executive summary component, 113; guidelines for, 58; internal assessment of, 38; prevalence of, 58–59

Moses Cone Health System, 198–199

N

National Cancer Center, website of, 36

National Center for Health Statistics, website of, 36

Nike, mission statement of, 62, 63

Nordstrom, strategy statement of, 72

Norton, David, 180, 185

Novant Health System, 198–199
Nurses, shortage of, 7, 21, 161

O

Objectives, 3; abandonment of, 119; for centers of excellence, 96; communication of, 20–21; definition of, 89; establishment of, 88–89; failure to implement, 15; identification of, 20; integration into implementation framework, 105; nonachievable, 119

Operating margin, 156, 157, 158

Operational benefits, of strategic planning, 152–153, 159–163, 167; case example of, 162–163; emergency department and ambulatory care flow, 160, 161; patient satisfaction, 159, 160, 161, 162; quality, 160, 161; staffing, 160, 161–162

Operational skills, *versus* strategic skills, 208–209

Operational thinking, differentiated from strategic thinking, 206–207

Opportunity testing, 197, 198

Organizational development departments, 133

Organizational direction, 8, 9, 10; development of, 60–61; example of, 114; identification of, 57–75; principle outputs of, 57, 58; purpose of, 9, 10; relationship to strategic thinking, 206; relationship to strategy formulation, 77, 78; updating of, 194

Organizational direction statements, development of, 60–61

Organization of Petroleum Exporting Countries (OPEC), 49

Orientation meetings, 29

Outcomes. *See also* Benefits: identification and communication of, 20–21

Outcomes-oriented statements, 20

Outpatient services, operational improvement of, 160, 161

Overall cost leadership strategy, 70

Overanalysis, 15, 20; of environmental assessment data, 35, 37; of historical data, 27, 37

P

Partnerships, between healthcare organizations and communities, 164, 165–166

Patient-centric healthcare, 21

Patient Protection and Affordable Care Act, 6–7

Patients, role in strategic planning, 146

Patient satisfaction: balanced scorecard assessment of, 181,

Simulation, 212

Sioux, 1

Situation analysis, 33. *See also* Environmental assessments

Society for Healthcare Strategy and Market Development, 227

Sony, 66, 208

Staff/staffing. *See also* Nurses; Physicians: internal assessment of, 39; operational improvement of, 160, 161–162, 163; shortages in, 160, 161–162

Stakeholders, involvement in strategic planning, 23–24, 139, 141–144, 145, 146; communication of strategic planning process to, 21–22; in strategic plan implementation, 173

Stanford University, vision statement of, 66

Strategic cycling model, 222, 224

Strategic management, 185–188; approaches to, 187–188; benefits of, 175–176, 185, 187; definition of, 186; relationship to strategic planning, 175–176, 185–187; stages of, 12

Strategic momentum, benefits of, 12

Strategic planners, new role of, 224–230

Strategic planning, 103-103. *See also* Environmental assess-ments; Implementation planning; Organizational direction; Preplanning steps; Strategy formula-tion: approaches to, 7–10; basic practices in, 227–228; best practices in, 227–230; bottom-up, 229; bottom-up *versus* top-down, 144, 149; contemporary *versus* past approaches in, 50; continuous, 147-148, 191. *See also* Annual strategic plan update; coordination of, 143; decentralized *versus* centralized, 147; definition of, 2–3, 79; description and communication of, 21–22; drawbacks to, 175, 209–210; duration of, 26; dynamic *versus* static, 230; effective, 31–32, 79–80, 132; with external orientation, 229; flexibility of, 147–148, 229; history of, 4, 5–6; key con-stituencies' involvement in, 139; linear *versus* nonlinear (iterative), 221–224; local or regional basis for, 5–6; major processes in, 131–149; narrative summary of, 121, 126–130; negative effects of, 1; in non-healthcare orga-nizations, 3–5, 227–230; nonlinear (iterative), 221–224; nonstrategic nature of, 4–5; obstacles to, 14–16; as

ongoing activity, 119; rationale for, 9, 10; relationship
to strategic management,
175–176, 185–187; relevance
of, 1–19; requirements for,
31–32; research approaches
in, 139–141; responsibility
for, 105; retreat planning
component of, 136–139;
strategic cycling model of,
222, 224; *versus* strategic
thinking, 208–212; successful, 32; survey of, 2; teamwork in, 135–136; time frame
for, 17; top-down, 229;
top-down *versus* bottom-up,
144, 149; use in the military,
2; work days required for, 5
Strategic planning committees, 24, 142; annual strategic plan updating role of,
196; disengagement from
strategic planning process,
88; goal identification role
of, 83, 85; implementation
monitoring role of, 119, 120;
implementation role of,
119–121, 173, 175; mission
statement development role
of, 63–64; senior manage-
ment members of, 45, 143;
strategic plan review and
updating role of, 113–114,
117, 119–121; strategic plan
review by, 113–114, 117;
teamwork by, 135

Strategic plans: adoption of,
111–118; alignment with pillars of excellence, 112, 115–
116; approval of, 117–118,
195; changes to, 13; com-
munication of, 103, 104; of
corporations, 5; cost of, 5;
customization of, 21–22;
distribution of, 113–114;
draft form of, 113–114, 117;
duration of, 118; manage-
ment action plan compo-
nent of, 88; new, approval
of, 195; nonapproval of, 118;
obsolescence of, 12–13; presentation of, 117–118; review
of, 105, 117–119; roll out
of, 104, 121, 174; strategy
component of, 88; successful, 13; tactical component
of, 88
Strategic skills, *versus* operational skills, 208–209
Strategic thinking, 205–220;
advanced, 217–220; benefits
of, 12; blue ocean strategy
of, 215–216; contingency
planning approach to, 212;
decision analysis approach
to, 214; definition of,
205–208; differentiated
from operational think-
ing, 206–207; game theory
approach to, 214; matrix of,
208–209; purposes of, 206;
scenario planning approach
to, 212–214; sensitivity

analysis approach to, 212; simulation approach to, 212; stimulation of, 29–31; *versus* strategic planning, 208–212

Stratego, 2

Strategy(ies): characteristics of, 71–72; cost leadership, 70; development of, 69–72; differentiated from operational effectiveness, 69; differentiation, 70–71; effective, 13–14; extrapolation of, 29–30; linear, 211; management tools *versus,* 59–60; merger, 7; mimicking of, 30; nonlinear, 211; past, review of, 28; performance failure of, 169–172

Strategy finders, 226

Strategy formulation, 9, 10, 77–92. *See also* Goals; Objectives: contingency planning component of, 89–90, 91; critical issues determination component of, 79–81; financial analysis component of, 90, 92; focus of, 194; goals identification component of, 78, 81, 83–88; implementation issues in, 173–174; initiatives identification output of, 78, 85–88; purpose of, 10; relationship to organizational direction, 77, 78; task force for, 82–88; updating of, 194–195

Strategy statements: examples of, 113; as executive summary component, 113

SurveyMonkey®, 140

Surveys, 2, 43, 140

Sustainability, of effective strategy, 13

SWOT (strengths, weaknesses/limitations, opportunities and threats), 34, 37–40, 46, 48

T

Task forces: for annual strategic plan updating, 196; for strategy formulation, 82–88

Teams, effective, 135–136

Teamwork, in strategic planning, 135–136

Telephone surveys, 43

Thinking. *See also* Strategic thinking: choice and consequences ("more/less"), 219; content ("either/or"), 219; creative, 31; holistic, 218; operational, 206–207

Thinking concepts, 218–219

Thinking skills, 217–218

Thinking styles, 219–220

Thinking techniques, 219

3M, mission statement of, 62, 63

"Tired of Strategic Planning" (Beinhocker and Kaplan), 211–212

To Err Is Human (Institute of Medicine), 161

Tools for Thinking Strategically (TTS), 217–220

Total quality management, 4

Transitioning to implementation, 103–130; executive summary component of, 111, 112–113, 114–116; key elements of, 103–105; monitoring and updating of strategic plans during, 118–121; strategic plan communication and roll out component of, 121–123; strategic plan review component of, 113–114, 117

Transparency, of information, 21

Trends analysis, 38; as external assessment component, 40–41, 43, 45

Walmart, 208
Wayne Memorial Health System, 85, 86
Welch, Jack, 4, 57

Z

Zero sum games, 215

About the Author

Alan M. Zuckerman, FACHE, FAAHC, is president of Health Strategies & Solutions, Inc., a healthcare strategy firm, and one of the nation's leading healthcare strategists. During his career, Mr. Zuckerman's consulting work has focused on strategic planning and competitive strategy; this book is an outgrowth of his experience with hundreds of diverse healthcare organizations, including many of the top hospitals, health systems, and academic medical centers in the country. Mr. Zuckerman is a frequent speaker on a variety of healthcare topics, the author of six books, and a winner of the ACHE's James A. Hamilton Award for book of the year.